Lecture Notes in Medical Informatics

Vol. 1: Medical Informatics Europe 78. Proceedings 1978. Edited by J. Anderson. XI, 822 pages. 1978.

Vol. 2: D. Fenna, S. Abrahamsson, S. O. Lööw and H. Peterson, The Stockholm County Medical Information System. VI, 163 pages. 1978.

Vol. 3: Long-Term Studies on Side-Effects of Contraception – State and Planning. Symposium 1977. Edited by U. Kellhammer and K. Überla. VI, 240 pages. 1978.

Vol. 4: Clinical Trials in 'Early' Breast Cancer. Proceedings 1978. Edited by H. R. Scheurlen, G. Weckesser and I. Armbruster. VI, 283 pages. 1979.

Vol. 5: Medical Informatics Berlin 1979. Proceedings 1979. Edited by B. Barber, F. Grémy, K. Überla and G. Wagner. XXIII, 970 pages. 1979.

Vol. 6: Health Care Technology Evaluation. Proceedings, 1978. Edited by J. Goldman. VII, 118 pages. 1979.

Vol. 7: Technology and Health: Man and his World. Proceedings, 1978. Edited by G. Wagner, P. L. Reichertz and E. Masè. VI, 243 pages. 1980.

Lecture Notes in Medical Informatics

Edited by D. A. B. Lindberg and P. L. Reichertz

7

Technology and Health: Man and his World

A SALUTIS UNITAS Contribution to an
International Conference on Medical
Informatics
Riva, del Garda, Italy, April 21–25, 1978

Edited by
G. Wagner, P. L. Reichertz, and E. Masè

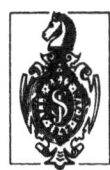

Springer-Verlag
Berlin Heidelberg New York 1980

Editors

Gustav Wagner
Institut für Dokumentation,
Information und Statistik
Deutsches Krebsforschungszentrum
Im Neuenheimer Feld 280
6900 Heidelberg 1
Germany

Peter L. Reichertz
Dept. für Biometrie und Dokumentation
Abt. für klinische Datenverarbeitung
und Dokumentation der Med. Hochschule
Karl-Wiechert-Allee 9
3000 Hannover 61
Germany

Ezio Masè
Via Tarvisio 5
I-00198 Roma
Italy

ISBN 978-3-540-10230-4   ISBN 978-3-642-49276-1(eBook)
DOI 10.1007/978-3-642-49276-1

2145/3140-543210

Foreword

SALUTIS UNITAS, Unity for Health, an organization 'Uniting physicians of the world to foster better health for all people through international exchange of technological information', was officially founded in 1972 after preceding years of preparation. One of its main objectives is the scientific communication, be it by meeting or by publications. So several scientific meetings could be held, mostly together with other scientific organizations, and resulted in the publication of the respective proceedings [1]. Studies were commissioned [2] to investigate trends in health care delivery and their socio-economic consequences, which also provided the basis for further investigations [3].

So also in 1978 an international congress was organized by SALUTIS UNITAS and sponsored by the international Menarini Foundation under its directorship of Dr. Gorini. This volume is based on the contributions of SALUTIS UNITAS members of this meeting 'Man and his World, Technology and Health', supplemented by further studies and materials.

The main objective was to look at various recipients of health care delivery: the individual, the community, the region and the nation. Emphasis was placed on systems analysis, simulation techniques and evaluation. According to the composition of the SALUTIS UNITAS membership, conceptual and interdisciplinary aspects prevail over descriptions of in-depth methodology, thus providing a broad access to the problems investigated.

For the Editors

---

1 Amongst others see: Masè, E., Collen, M.F., Gorini, S. (Eds): The Computer in Health Care Systems in Some European Countries and in the United States (Piccin, Padua 1976).

2 Chadwick, J.H.: Health Service Systems for a Finite World. Salutis Unitas Report (Stanford Research Institute, Project 3595, Menlo Park/USA 1975).

3 E.g.: Reichertz, P.L., Anderson, J.: A Systems View of Health Care Organizations. In: Laudet, M., Anderson, J., Begon, F. (Eds): Medical Computing, pp. 87-98 (Taylor and Francis, London 1977).

Table of Contents

Introductory Address

E. Masè

In the incessant struggle waged by man for supremacy in the world
around him, he has succeeded in continuously modifying the earth by
modifications often no less relevant than those caused by geographical
and physical factors. It is, therefore, in a geographical and anthro-
pological perspective that the great epic of human labor is best seen,
an epic which had its beginnings many millennia ago, but undoubtedly
is still not completed, if we think in terms of insuring the survival
of the species.

The signs of man's intervention made their appearance from the time
he gradually began to people the vast spaces of the earth. These
migrations were made possible by the extraordinary physiological
capacity of man to adapt to the most varied and extreme conditions
obtaining in the furthermost longitudes and latitudes of the globe.
In this process, man began to realize that his life does not only
consist of himself, but also of the world around him, especially when
the original microcurrent of migration swelled into macrocurrents of
human displacement all over the globe.

In the flow of these migratory currents, man first circulates under
the pressure of natural events, then under the impulse of the most
varied motives which can be summed up as economic and commercial,
socio-cultural, religious, and even health-related. Mingling together
in a lively fashion - not a few times with furore - these movements
make the great river of history flow. It is a river which, as it
irrigates the length and breadth of the planet, produces the thoughts
and works of the various civilizations of man. In passing, we note
that in this perspective we find the confirmation of the theory that
geography alone does not determine history, but undoubtedly
influences it.

The relation of man with his world, as he comes to dominate it more
and more through his prodigious scientific and technological capacity,
can be validly summarized in the sentence of the Spanish philosopher
Ortega y Gasset: "I am myself and my circumstances". Here the close
link between history and geography is made clearly evident. In fact,

circumstances are obviously correlated to man at a given position in space and at a particular moment in time. These circumstances, however, do not completely condition his behaviour, since he is free, according to his intellectual and physical capacities, to choose among the various possibilities offered by circumstances.

The wisdom of these choices over the course of the centuries reveals itself to be in direct proportion to the quantity and quality of information collected about man himself and his environment. It is only the most knowledgeable choices that have enabled man to realize himself most effectively and brought him into close contact with his world.

But the most binding contact between man and his world is created when, as today, more knowledgeable choices can be obtained with the aid of the computer, the most significant instrument that technology has ever produced for further cultural evolution. In fact, a far greater dominion over the play of "circumstances" inherent in the quality of life now becomes possible.

Continuing in this geographical-historical perspective, we can now turn to what presents itself as the most relevant of all circumstances in the relation between man and his world, namely illness. In fact, this has constituted a serious menace to his survival from the most ancient times, all the more so, when accompanied by famine and war. The biblical invocation in this regard goes back to the pre-history of man, especially following the tremendous epidemics that have in their time repeatedly devastated the world.

Only in the 15th century did these catastrophes enable the medical geographer Paracelsus to intuit the dynamic essence of illness. This concept gradually developed and found scientific confirmation when, as today, the state of illness is being interpreted as a consequence of complex interactions between the human organism and the environment.

If we consider health as the highest social value, because of the benefits the entire human society derives from it, then the actualization of health care delivery systems which assure in the best way the protection of health becomes a problem of primary importance. Originating in still recent times for groups of working people and then gradually becoming more and more extensive, many of these systems entered into a crisis, now more than ever aggravated by the escalation of chronic and degenerative illnesses, as well as by multiple environmental pollution.

Because of the explosion of costs and the consequent degradation of
the quality of health services, this crisis now afflicts all Western
countries, independent of their political systems and independent of
the social methods operating at the base of the systems themselves.
The basic cause of this crisis must, therefore, be considered as
prevalently structural and managerial in character.

We must bear in mind that the productivity of any system today is
totally tied to the presence of the computer which provides for the
automatic elaboration of data and information flowing into it from
the nodal points of the system itself.

Analogously, an efficient health care delivery system needs the
computer as the basic instrument of medical informatics, the new
discipline that has recently come into being in response to the need
for applying the very concept of "system" to medicine, considered
both as a science and as an instrument of health care.

By undertaking to document, analyze, direct, control and summarize
the informative processes of medicine, this new discipline has
rendered possible that continuous, precise and accurate exchange of
information between those preventive, diagnostic, therapeutic and
rehabilitative sectors absolutely indispensable to the doctor for a
more exact evaluation of the state of health or illness.

The introduction of medical technology into health care delivery
systems could not fail to arouse a certain diffidence, just as every
innovation has done in the past, in our case principally because
operating costs were considered too high. Then, there is the
objection to a presumed de-humanization or even the destruction of
many traditional values, including that represented by the doctor-
patient relationship.

These as well as other negative judgments are, however, considered
to be superseded by the facts successively established. In reality,
the costs of operating the present systems have become insupportable
in practice. Vast state expenditures feed the area of health services
in a disorderly fashion and with scarce productivity.

The doctor-patient relationship has likewise undergone considerable
erosion in the process, because of the restricted time any doctor
can on the average devote to a patient in the framework of the
present systems.

In contrast, experience so far has clearly demonstrated the high
degree of efficiency, availability and productivity that can be

reached by health services when they are adequately equipped with the instruments of modern medical technology. In fact, the development of automatized systems has demonstrated their ability to bring about a positive revolution in all phases of health care as well as an increase in the availability of time at the disposition of the doctor for his patient. In all phases and at every level, thanks to this technological progress, health protection can now be extended to every environmental level, from the individual through the rural, urban, regional and up to the national level, with consequently greater contact between man and his world.

Our present epoch, therefore, is one of great expectations, and of no lesser demands for increased health protection. In point of fact, public opinion and the press are exerting more and more pressure on legislators for health systems capable of overcoming a crisis situation that is becoming more and more serious, more costly, and of long duration.

The wind of change is blowing with greater intensity and insistence in this direction in many countries, including Italy, where a health reform bill is even now under discussion in Parliament. It is high time - and politicians should be more sensitive to this situation - for an out and out technological confrontation between the old and the new.

The present moment in the history of the health services might well find symbolic expression in a painting I had occasion to admire recently in an art gallery. I do not recall the name of this picture, but its title might well have been "The day everything changed". The canvas, in fact, depicted a race between an automobile and a horse, and the artist caught the scene at the moment when the car was just about to pass the horse. An attentive crowd is watching the contest between horse and machine very closely. Although the painting gives no indication of time or place, we know for certain that this race will be won by the automobile.

It is a victory which made global distances shrink further and brought about a further extension of man's dominion over his environment. Our painting indeed showed us "A day when everything changed" because of a confrontation that had to come. And, in fact, a technology and a way of life, not merely of an entire country, but of the whole world had changed for ever.

It is now abundantly clear that, as regards the protection of health, we are living a "Day" likewise destined to be an epoch of transition which similarly develops through the various stages of an equally inevitable confrontation.

As these stages succeed one another, they can, however, be subject to delays, as in fact has already happened. However, further delays would be without sufficiently valid motivation, since they tend to keep man in an area ecologically more and more dangerous for his survival.

As governments more and more find themselves prisoners of the suffocating spiral of health costs, the individual and the communities at their various levels also remain prisoners of the consequent degradation of the health services, and this in an epoch of prodigious development of medicine and medical technology, that is to say, just at the moment when man can begin to make use of health care delivery systems which render possible a valid control of illness according to objectives definable a priori in terms of costs and services. This control reduces the frequency of the "circumstances" of the illness and in doing so concedes greater liberty of choice to man and, thereby, greater realization of himself.

Salutis Unitas has been battling for almost a decade against these delays in the adoption of advanced technology in health care delivery systems. The authors of the contributions in this book who are all members of Salutis Unitas are discussing various applications of these new technologies, methods and systems, many of which, be it noted, could already be introduced into existing health services.

This will render evident that the extensive development of a universal instrument like the computer is capable not only of forging more productive, efficient and accessible health care systems, but also of rendering the decisional capacity of the doctor more informed and rational with resultant greater prestige and dignity for him.

Periodic Health Examinations of Individuals

M.F. Collen

Introduction

Personal preventive services in primary medical care are based to
some extent upon periodic re-evaluation of the health status of
the individual. Such health examinations (health evaluations,
health appraisals or health checkups) are usually initiated by the
patient; but they may result from the recommendation of a physician,
a commercial company (6, 29, 45), a health care program (40) or
a public health agency (35, 59).

The traditional method in the USA for a patient to obtain a health
examination is to see a primary care physician, who takes a medical
history from the patient, provides a physical examination and then
arranges for diagnostic tests and procedures which in the
physician's judgment are necessary to complete the health
evaluation. The physician then makes a determination as to whether
the patient is well or sick and recommends appropriate followup
care (1).

Multiphasic Health Testing (MHT) is a systemized approach to
providing the laboratory testing portion of a health examination
and it employs automated laboratory procedures and specially
trained allied health personnel to collect data on patients' medical
histories, clinical laboratory, x-ray and other physiological test
measurements in a programmed sequence (20, 21). MHT is followed by
a physical examination provided by a physician who decides if the
patient is well or sick, and then recommends appropriate followup
care (7,10,15,67).

MHT developed from the experience of public health mass screening
(2, 3, 50, 69, 73, 74), which was modified in order to furnish
personal preventive medical services to meet the needs of individual
patients and their physicians (63, 68). Over the past 45 years,
MHT evolved as a systemized approach to provide health examinations

more efficiently to large groups (2). The concept of health checkups is not new, as for decades the practice of periodic health examinations has been recommended generally. In order to decrease the costs of providing such examinations, some of the principles and methods of systems engineering have been applied in multiphasic health testing (23). There was a gradual evolution through the various historical steps of screening, mass screening, multiphasic screening, automated multiphasic screening, multiphasic health testing to the most advanced automated multiphasic health testing services (43, 64). MHT programs are now widespread throughout the developed countries of the world. At the present time, there are about 300 in the U.S.A., about 50 in Japan, about 30 in Europe, and a few in Australia, Asia, Canada and Latin America (16, 61).

Objectives of Health Examinations

The usual purposes of providing health examinations are:

1. Provide reassurance, since many patients who come to see their physicians for a health examination are worried about their health.

2. Define the health status of examinees and determine individual fitness (health appraisal); monitor the status of the continuing health of individuals by periodic examinations (health surveillance).

3. Detect unknown abnormalities (disease detection or case finding); monitor previously detected abnormalities by the periodic examination of patients with known diabetes, hypertension, etc. (patient surveillance and disease monitoring).

4. Serve as an entry mode to a health care system; provide hospital pre-admission examinations.

5. Provide health education and health maintenance to improve health habits and behavior.

6. Provide a comprehensive, good quality, patient "health profile" to furnish baseline measurements for continuing or future care.

7. Improve the outcome of patients by decreasing morbidity, disability and mortality.

Test Selection for Health Problems

It is important to identify a set of health conditions, tests and
preventive procedures for each program of health examinations, to
fit the needs of its target population (4, 5, 60, 66, 72). It is
advisable to have a somewhat different battery of tests for young,
middle-aged and older adults.

1. Selecting Conditions for Testing

Important health problems for the individual include not only
conditions which are potentially disabling or life-threatening
(e.g., hypertension, breast cancer (25), etc.), but conditions
which impair the quality of life (e.g., anxiety, impaired hearing,
etc.). Each condition should be sufficiently prevalent in the
population tested and have a test available to detect the
condition with sufficient sensitivity and specificity so that the
cost per positive test is acceptable to both the provider and
user of services. In other words, the predicted yield rate in the
target population must be appreciable; if the condition is rare, it
will probably be too expensive to detect.

Appropriate health care services should be available for the condition, whether this be further diagnostic, curative or rehabilitative services, health and psychosocial counseling, or palliative
care - as may be indicated for each patient's problem (19, 71).
It is ideal (but not always achievable in reality) if the test can
detect the disease early enough, and if effective therapy is
available, such that the entire process of detection, diagnosis
and treatment can be demonstrated to be cost-effective.

2. Specific Test Selection

The test must be acceptable to the patient; it must be harmless,
cause no unreasonable discomfort and take a reasonable length of
time.

The cost per test must be acceptable to patients as a reasonable
charge (65). The cost per positive test (18) is basic to test
selection, and is the result of the cost per test (17), the test
sensitivity, and the prevalence of the condition in the target
population (70).

Using a cost analysis for the Kaiser-Permanente program, the MHT costs for a representative test (chest x-ray) will be considered as an example. Table 1 shows the cost per positive for three tests, for

Table 1: Cost per Positive Test by Age Group

Test	Under 40		40 - 59		60 & Over	
	%+	$/+	%+	$/+	%+	$/+
Blood Pressure	0.4	88	4.3	8	11.5	3
E.K.G.	10.2	9	17.7	5	31.5	3
Chest X-ray	2.1	69	7.4	20	19.2	8

(Modified from reference [18])

young, middle-aged and older persons (18). The unit cost for a chest x-ray (including all direct and indirect costs and the radiologist's interpretation) was $ 1.45. Only clinically important abnormalities were included, since the definition of "abnormal" is critical in establishing yield rates and unit costs. Table 1 shows for chest x-rays the tenfold increase in frequency of clinically important abnormalities reported in adults over age 60, as compared to those under age 40. The unit cost per positive chest x-ray for a clinically important abnormality in the 60 years and older age group was only $ 8. The low prevalence and high unit cost per positive test for chest x-rays for young adults has caused some MHT programs to omit chest x-rays for this group.

It must be emphasized that these low unit costs for Kaiser-Permanente were related to an MHT patient load of about 2,000 examinations per month at that time. If only 1,000 persons were examined monthly, the cost per patient would probably double. If 3,000 persons could be tested per month, the unit cost would probably decrease by about one third. These data clearly demonstrate how the prevalence of an abnormal test is dependent upon age composition of the specific population examined. It is also important to emphasize that,in order to evaluate the true efficiency of any test for case detection, it requires an extension of the analysis to determine the cost per proven "true" positive case, which requires expensive followup confirmatory and validating procedures.

Evaluation of Periodic Health Examinations

Periodic health examinations, to be properly evaluated, must be studied to determine to what extent they are effective in decreasing mortality and disability and to attempt to measure their cost benefits (8, 9, 31-38, 44-49, 51-58, 62, 75).

1. Effect on Mortality of Urging Multiphasic Checkups

The most important objective of periodic health checkups is to decrease morbidity and mortality. The only long-term randomized clinical trial, a controlled study of the effect of urging adults to have annual multiphasic health checkups, has been conducted over the past ten years by the Kaiser-Permanente Medical Care Program (30-32, 39).

From a pool of 46,000 eligible Kaiser Foundation Health Plan members, ages 35-54, two groups were randomly selected. The "study" group of 5,156 members has been urged to have a multiphasic health checkup every year. The "control" group of 5,557 members has been left alone. Both groups have been followed up in identical fashion to assess mortality.

The major mortality findings are summarized in Table 2.

Table 2: Deaths and Death Rates in Study and Control Group Subjects, 1965-73

	Number of Deaths[*]		Death Rate (per 1000 for 9 yrs.)		Chi Square Value
	Study	Control	Study	Control	
Potentially postponable causes	35	59	6.8	10.7	4.51[**]
Cancer of colon & rectum	3	14	0.6	2.5	6.34[**]
Cancer of breast (women only)	12	11	4.3	3.8	0.10
Cancer of cervix & uterus	0	2	0.0	0.7	0.46
Cancer of prostate (men only)	0	1	0.0	0.4	0.00
Hypertension, hypertensive cardio-vascular dis., & hypertensive hemorrhagic cerebrovascular dis.	10	22	2.0	4.0	3.65
Hemorrhagic cerebrovascular dis. without hypertension	9	9	1.8	1.6	0.00
Other Causes	240	247	46.7	44.6	0.27
All Causes	275	306	53.5	55.3	0.16

[*] Populations alive as of January 1, 1965; Study-5156, Control-5557; [**] $p < .05$.

The death rate through 1973 has been significantly lower in the study group for conditions hypothesized in advance to be detectable by checkups and amenable to therapy that would prevent or postpone mortality. For the nine years, the death rate for these potentially postponable conditions (largely the accessible cancers and hypertensive disease) has been 6.8/1000 in the study group, based on 35 deaths, and 10.7/1000 in the control group, based on 59 deaths (p < .05). The two conditions chiefly responsible for the study-control difference in mortality were hypertension and colorectal cancer.

Although the overall mortality rates from all causes are similar for the study and the control groups (see Table 2), an interesting observation has been made that in the entire population of 10,713 persons there is a gradient risk of mortality from all causes according to the number of checkups the subjects have received, whether in the study or control group. The mortality rates and age-standardized mortality ratios for all causes of death in all subjects are shown in Table 3. The mortality rates were calculated

Table 3: Mortality Rates and Standard Mortality Ratios,
all Subjects, 1965-73

No. of MHT's 1965-73	Person-Years of observation in this category	Number of deaths	Crude mortality rate(deaths/1000 person-years)	Standard. mortality ratio
0	38,384	310	8.08	1.38
1	19,039	112	5.88	1.02
2	11,189	51	4.56	0.74
3	7,874	36	4.57	0.71
4-6	13,282	59	4.44	0.62
7+	3,959	13	3.28	0.40

on a person-year basis in such a way that having more checkups was not confounded with survival. It has been determined that serious illness at the start of the study was not responsible for this mortality gradient. Obviously, in departing from comparison of the study and control groups and comparing different degrees of cooperation of use of checkups, the bias of self-selection can become important. The characteristics of the low and high utilizers of checkups have not yet been compared to determine the extent to which the mortality gradient can be explained by the effects of

self-selection. The mortality differences attributable to
checkups are thus overstated in Table 3, whereas in the study vs.
control group comparison (Table 2) they are understated due to the
effect of crossovers between the two groups. A true measure of the
effect of checkups on mortality probably is somewhere between
the figures shown in Tables 2 and 3.

On the basis of these studies, periodic health examinations are
recommended every 1-2 years for the middle-aged and elderly, and
less often for younger persons.

2. Cost-Benefits of MHT

A limited cost-benefit study of periodic health examinations using
MHT has been conducted at Kaiser-Permanente Oakland and San
Francisco which measured its effect on disability, mortality and
the earnings of non-disabled survivors (16, 22, 28, 56). In this
project, a "study" group of approximately 1,229 men who were
Kaiser Health Plan members, initially ages 45-54, were urged to
undertake annual MHT examinations. A "control" group of similar
composition and size were not so urged but were followed up in a
similar fashion for each subject's health experience. The group
described herein constitutes the one age-sex subgroup in whom a
favorable effect on disability was found.

Expenses associated with health-related events were compiled for
the study and control groups. Medical care utilization was
measured in the study and control group subjects in the Health
Plan. Disability rates were measured in subjects who remained in
the Kaiser Plan and responded to mailed questionnaires. Self-rated
disability has limitations but does provide some measure of
health status.

Table 4 depicts the net difference in earnings in the study and

Table 4: Cost-Benefit Analysis of Periodic MHT Examinations in Men (Ages 45-54 at Entry)

		1965	1966	1967	1968	1969	1970	1971	1965-1971 Total
Percent of initial group with no or partial disability									
1. No disability	C	86.8	83.9	81.0	78.6	76.2	73.1	70.1	
	S	87.5	85.5	83.2	82.2	81.2	77.8	74.2	
2. Partial disability	C	10.4	11.4	12.5	13.3	14.0	15.2	16.4	
	S	10.3	11.1	11.9	11.2	10.6	11.3	12.1	
Average annual earnings/man	C	$7038	$7132	$7350	$7850	$8271	$8678	$9270	
	S	$7083	$7234	$7488	$8036	$8510	$8863	$9371	
Average earnings difference/man	S-C	$45	$102	$138	$186	$239	$185	$101	$996
Net difference after deducting MHT & Clinic expense	S-C	$41	$78	$113	$157	$210	$155	$68	$822

S = Study group of 1,229 men (in 1965) urged to have a MHT examination every year.
C = Control group of 1,364 men (in 1965) not so urged, but voluntarily could obtain such exams.

(Modified from references [16,22]).

control groups. The first four rows contain the proportions of survivors with no or partial disability adjusted to relate to the initial population, so as to account for additional losses in earnings due to mortality. "No disability" was defined in the survey questionnaire as a present state of health enabling one to do one's usual work with no limitation. "Partial disability" was de- fined as a present state of health which caused one to limit or cut down on the amount or kind of work one was doing.

The combined proportions of living men with no disability and partial disability were multiplied by annual income estimates to give the average annual earnings per man in the initial populations. The study-control group differences represent the differences in average annual earnings due to differences in disability prevalence and mortality per man in the initial populations.

The study-control group differences in net earnings, after deduct- ing the MHT expenses and additional outpatient clinic expenses, are shown in the last row. It can be seen that the total economic impact favored the study group every year. The total difference for the 7-year period is over $ 800 per man. It can therefore be

concluded that urging 45-54 year old men to have an MHT
examination every year has important cost-benefits. It should also
be pointed out that the amount of   savings associated with
greater MHT exposure applied to men in the middle income range,
who formed the majority of the subjects in this study. For men with
higher incomes the difference would be greater; for men with lower
incomes it would be less. The study did not demonstrate, however,
that multiphasic health checkups provided similar cost-benefits for
other groups, such as 35-44 year old males or 35-54 year old
females.

Evaluation of Alternative Health Examination Modes

If it is necessary to respond to the public's demand for periodic
health examinations, or if an organizational decision is made to
provide health examinations to a group of people, the question
arises as to which is the most cost-effective examination method.
The following study compared, for two similar groups of patients
"new" to the doctor, the costs of health examinations provided by
MHT to health examinations provided in a traditional way by
physicians (24-27, 41, 42).

In the Kaiser-Permanente Oakland Medical Center, one group of
1,916 patients received a MHT, followed by a 15-minute scheduled
visit for a physical examination by a physician in the medical
department (the MHT group). A comparable group of 2,040 patients
received a "traditional" medical checkup (the TMC group) provided
by the same physicians who, during a 30-minute scheduled visit,
took a history and did a physical examination. After the physician
saw the patient in either mode, he would refer the patient to
appropriate specialty clinics for "followup" clinical laboratory
tests, x-rays, EKG's and other special diagnostic procedures as
necessary to arrive at a final diagnosis.

All data were adjusted so that both groups were comparable by age,
sex and health status. Since the same physicians provided the
examinations and arranged followup care for both groups, the
quality of care was assumed to be similar. Table 5 shows the use

Table 5: Comparative Use and Cost of Services (Initial and Followup) for a Health
Examination (Adjusted for Age, Sex and Health Status)

	Initial Examination				Followup Services				Total Costs	
	TMC*		MHT**)		TMC		MHT		TMC	MHT
	No.	$	No.	$	No.	$	No.	$	$	$
Medical Dept. M.D. (min.)	30.0	28.52	15.0	14.75	12.2	9.39	8.7	5.61	37.91	20.36
Other Depts. M.D. (min.)	-	-	-	-	1.4	1.43	1.8	1.84	1.43	1.84
MHT	0	0	1	17.46	-	-	-	-	0	17.46
Clinical Lab. (tests)	6.45	10.71	0	0	3.14	5.21	1.48	2.45	15.92	2.45
X-ray (films)	0.87	3.60	0	0	0.31	1.27	0.38	1.57	4.87	1.57
ECG, etc.	0.13	0.71	0	0	0.10	0.58	0.20	1.12	1.29	1.12
Total	$43.54		$32.21		$17.88		$12.59		$61.42	$44.80

*) TMC = 2,040 persons   **) MHT = 1,916 persons   (Modified from references [16,26]).

and cost of services for the initial examination visit by the two
modes. The costs shown are expenses to the Kaiser Health Plan for
the services provided to its members, and do not represent fees
or charges which would have been paid by non-member patients. The
MHT panel of tests replaced the individually selected tests which
were ordered by the physicians in the traditional mode. The great
decrease in physician time for the MHT initial physical
examination was obviously the main saving.

Table 5 also shows the followup visits and tests ordered by the
physicians to complete the health examination. Many patients did
not have their health examination fully completed at the initial
visit since the evaluation of possible variations from normal
required further diagnostic tests (clinical laboratory, radiology,
ECG, etc.) and/or physician specialist consultation visits (internal
medicine, ophthalmology, gynecology, dermatology, etc.) to confirm
the validity of the finding or the need for further diagnostic
evaluation. The costs for ancillary services (clinical laboratory,

radiology, ECG and other diagnostic procedures) used for the followup evaluation workups are also shown. The impact of the more comprehensive initial testing of MHT is shown here by comparing the sum of clinical laboratory + radiology + special diagnostic procedures for followup evaluations ($ 7.06 for TMC and $ 5.14 for MHT).

The total physician time (initial and followup), represented by scheduled minutes, was very different. The traditional (TMC) examination method used a total of 43.6 minutes of M.D. time on the average. The MHT mode reduced the physician time used in the initial examination by one half, and decreased somewhat the physician time used for followup evaluation, so that the average total was only 25.5 minutes, or 42 percent less M.D. time.

The total cost for a health examination is the sum of the resources used on the initial examination visit and on the evaluation followup visits. The average total cost for a health examination by the traditional (TMC) physician mode was $ 61.42. By first providing a MHT battery of tests, followed by a physician physical examination, the total costs for a health examination were decreased to $ 44.80 (for a decrease in total costs of 27 percent). Since the total costs for ancillary tests (MHT, clinical laboratory, x-ray and ECG) were similar for both modes (about $ 22), the cost differences were entirely due to saving of physician time.

Of additional importance was the finding that the initial increased comprehensiveness of the MHT examination, when serving as the entry mode to a health care system, had a significant economic impact on the subsequent followup care for at least one year.

Table 6 compares the total resource costs utilized per 1,000

Table 6: Summary of 12-Month Total Resource Costs
($/YR/1000 Examinees, Adjusted for Age,
Sex and Health Status)

	TMC	MHT
MD Costs (% of Traditional)	93,673 (100)	68,714 (73)
Total Costs (% of Traditional)	131,179 (100)	105,966 (81)

(Modified from reference [27]).

patients for 12 months beginning with the health examination. These costs include all physicians plus all supporting personnel, overhead and facilities' costs, etc. Patients who received the MHT examination saved $ 25,213 per 1,000 patients per year as compared to those who received a traditional medical checkup (TMC). The total cost of care for the MHT group over 12 months was 19 percent less than for the TMC group, primarily due to saving in physicians' time.

References

1. American Medical Association: A Manual of Suggestions for the Conduct of Periodic Examinations of Apparently Healthy Persons. Chicago 1925.

2. Breslow, L.: Multiphasic Screening Examinations - An Extension of the Mass Screening Technique. Amer.J.publ.Hlth 40 (1950) 274-278.

3. Breslow, L.: Historical Review of Multiphasic Screening. Prev.Med. 2 (1973) 1977-196.

4. Breslow, L., et al.: Theory, Practice and Application of
   Prevention in Personal Health Services. In Preventive Medicine
   USA. Prodist, New York 1976.

5. Breslow, L., Sommers, A.R.: The Lifetime Health-Monitoring
   Program. New Engl.J.Med. 296 (1977) 601-608.

6. Burr, H.B.: Westinghouse Management Health Examinations and
   Their Investment Value. J.occup.Med. 2 (1960) 80-91.

7. Caceres, C.: AMHT in Perspective - Accomplishments and Problems.
   In Automated Multiphasic Health Testing. Engineering Foundation
   Research Conferences. Engineering Foundation, New York 1971.

8. Cochrane, A.L., Holland, W.W.: Validation of Screening
   Procedures. Bri.med.Bull. 25 (1971) 3-8.

9. Cochrane, A.L.: Effectiveness and Efficiency: Random Reflections
   on Health Services. Nuffield Provincial Hospital Trust,
   London 1972.

10. Collen, F.B., Madero, B., Soghikian, K., Garfield, S.R.: Kaiser-
    Permanente Experiment in Ambulatory Care. Amer.J.Nurs. 71
    (1971) 1371-1374.

11. Collen, M.F., Linden, C.: Screening in a Group Practice Prepaid
    Medical Care Plan. J.chron.Dis. 2 (1955) 400-406.

12. Collen, M.F., Rubin, L., Neyman, J., Dantzig, G., Baer, R.M.,
    Siegelaub, A.B.: Automated Multiphasic Screening and Diagnosis.
    Amer.J.publ.Hlth 54 (1964) 741-750.

13. Collen, M.F.: Multiphasic Screening as a Diagnostic Method in
    Preventive Medicine. Meth.Inform.Med. 4 (1965) 71-74.

14. Collen, M.F.: Periodic Health Examinations Using an Automated
    Multi-Test Laboratory. J.Amer.med.Ass. 195 (1966) 830-833.

15. Collen, M.F.: The Multitest Laboratory in Health Care of the
    Future. Hospitals 41 (1967) 119-122.

16. Collen, M.F. (Edit): Multiphasic Health Testing Services.
    John Wiley and Sons, New York 1978.

17. Collen, M.F., Kidd, P.H., Feldman, R.F., Cutler, J.L.: Cost Analysis of a Multiphasic Screening Program. New Engl.Med. 280 (1969) 1043-1045.

18. Collen, M.F., Feldman, R., Siegelaub, A.B., Crawford, D.: Dollar Cost per Positive Test for Automated Multiphasic Screening. New Engl.J.Med. 283 (1970) 459-463.

19. Collen, M.F.: Diseases Which Can and should Be Detected Early. Industr.Med. 39 (1970) 27-29.

20. Collen, M.F.: Implementation of a AMHT System. Hospitals 45 (1971) 49-58.

21. Collen, M.F.: Guidelines for Multiphasic Health Checkup. Arch. intern.Med. 127 (1971) 99-100.

22. Collen, M.F., Dales, L.G., Friedman, G.D., Flagle, C.D., Feldman, R., Siegelaub, A.B.: Multiphasic Checkup Evaluation Study: 4. Preliminary Cost Benefit Analysis for Middle-Aged Men. Prev.Med. 2 (1973) 236-246.

23. Collen, M.F.: Multiphasic Testing as a Triage to Medical Care. In Ingelfinger, F.J., Relman, A.S., Finland, M. (Eds): Controversy in Internal Medicine, Vol. 2, pp. 85-91. W.B. Saunders Co., Philadelphia 1974.

24. Collen, M.F., Garfield, S.R.: New Medical Care Delivery System, Final Report. January, 1975. National Technical Information Service (NTIS), Springfield, Va. P.B. 246 630.

25. Collen, M.F.: A Case Study of Mammography. Committee on Technology and Health Care. Nat.Acad.Sci., Washington, D.C. 1977.

26. Collen, M.F., Garfield, S.R., Richart, R.H., Duncan, J.H., Feldman, R.: Cost Analyses of Alternative Health Examination Modes. Arch.intern.Med. 137 (1977) 73-79.

27. Collen, M.F.: Cost Analysis of the Kaiser Foundation's Systemized Health Evaluation. In Preventive Medicine USA, pp. 707-714. Prodist, New York 1976.

28. Collen, M.F.: Systems Evaluation of MHTS. In Collen, M.F.
    (Edit.): Multiphasic Health Testing Services. John Wiley and
    Sons, New York 1978.

29. Collings, G.H., Jr., Dupong, W.G., Fitzpatrick, M.M., Frederick,
    W.S., Levy, B.F., Scott, M.R., Stratton, K.L., Walsh, J.M.,
    Wood, L.W., Zaves, N.A.: Multiphasic Health Screening in
    Industry. J.occup.Med. 14 (1972) 437-496.

30. Cutler, J.L., Ramcharan, S., Feldman, R., Siegelaub, A.,
    Campbell, B., Friedman, G.D., Dales, L.G., Collen, M.F.:
    Multiphasic Checkup Evaluation Study: 1. Methods and Population.
    Prev.Med. 2 (1973) 197-206.

31. Dales, L.G., Friedman, G.D., Ramcharan, S., Siegelaub, A.B.,
    Campbell, B.A., Feldman, R., Collen, M.F.: Multiphasic Checkup
    Evaluation Study: 3.Outpatient Clinic Utilization, Hospitali-
    zation and Mortality Experience after Seven Years. Prev.Med. 2
    (1973) 221-235.

32. Dales, L.G., Friedman, G.D., Collen, M.F.: Evaluation of a
    Periodic Multiphasic Health Checkup. Meth.Inform.Med. 12
    (1974) 140-146.

33. Deniston, O.L., Rosenstock, I.M., Getting, V.A.: Evaluation of
    Program Effectiveness. Publ.Hlth Rep. 83 (1968) 323-335.

34. Deniston, O.L., Rosenstock, I.M., Welch, W., Getting, V.A.:
    Evaluation of Program Efficiency. Publ.Hlth Rep. 83 (1968)
    603-610.

35. Detection and Prevention of Chronic Disease Utilizing Multiphasic
    Health Screening Techniques. Hearings before the Subcommittee
    on Health of the Elderly of the Special Committee on Aging,
    U.S.Senate. Sept. 1966.

36. Emlet, H.E.: A Preliminary Exploration of Cost Benefits for
    Multiphasic Health Screening. Presented at Engineering
    Foundation Research Conference in Engineering in Medicine.
    Multiphasic Screening III. Deerfield, Mass. 1969.

37. Flagle, C.D.: Automated Multiphasic Health Testing and Services.
Total Systems Analysis and Design. Meth.Inform.Med. 10 (1971)
201-206.

38. Flagle, C.D.: Evaluation and Control of Technology in Health
Services. In Collen, M.F. (Edit.): Technology and Health Care
Systems in the 1980's. DHEW Publ.No. (HSM) 73-3016, 1972.
U.S. Govt.Print.Off., Washington, D.C.

39. Friedman, G.D.: Effects of MHTS on Patients. In Collen, M.F.
(Edit.): Multiphasic Health Testing Services. John Wiley and
Sons, New York 1978.

40. Garfield, S.R.: Multiphasic Health Testing and Medical Care as
a Right. New Engl.J.Med. 283 (1970) 1087-1089.

41. Garfield, S.R.: The Delivery of Medical Care. Sci.Amer. 222
(1970) 15-23.

42. Garfield, S.R., Collen, M.F., Richart, R.H., Feldman, R.,
Soghikian, K., Duncan, J.H.: Evaluation of a New Ambulatory
Medical Care Delivery System. New Engl.J.Med. 294 (1976) 426-431.

43. Gelman, A.C.: Multiphasic Health Testing Systems: Reviews and
Annotations. H.E.W. Health Services and Mental Health Adm.
HSRD 71-1, 1971.

44. Grant, J.A.: Quantitative Evaluation of a Screening Program.
Amer.J.publ.Hlth 64 (1974) 66-70.

45. Grimaldi, J.V.: The Worth of Occupational Health Programs. A
New Evaluation of Periodic Physical Examinations. J.occup.Med.
7 (1965) 365-373.

46. Hill, A.B.: Principles of Medical Statistics, pp. 201-210.
9th Ed. Oxford University Press, Oxford 1971.

47. Holland, W.W.: Screening for Disease. Taking Stock. Lancet 1974,
II: 1494-1497.

48. Klarman, H.E.: Present Status of Cost-Benefit Analysis in the
Health Field. Amer.J.publ.Hlth 57 (1967) 1948-1953.

49. Klarman, H.E.: Application of Cost-Benefit Analysis to Health Systems Technology. In Collen, M.F. (Edit.): Technology and Health Care Systems in the 1980's, pp. 115-150. DHEW Publ.No. (HSM) 73-3016, 1972. U.S. Govt.Print.Off., Washington, D.C.; also in J.occup.Med. 16 (1974) 172-186.

50. Mass Health Examination as a Public Health Tool. Technical Report No. A24. Geneva, W.H.O. 1971.

51. McKeown, T.: Validation of Screening Procedures. In Nuffield Provincial Hospital Trust (Edit.): Screening in Medical Care. Oxford University Press, London 1968.

52. McKeown, T.: Validation of Screening. In Nuffield Provincial Hospital Trust (Edit.): Screening in Medical Care. Oxford University Press, London 1968.

53. Oszustowicz, R.J.: An Economic and Operational Analysis of Automated Health Testing and Screening in a Community Hospital. Proceedings of the Symposium of the International Health Evaluation Association, 1971.

54. Phillips, R.M., Hughes, J.P.: Cost Benefit Analysis of the Occupational Health Program: A Generic Model. J.occup.Med. 16 (1974) 158-161.

55. Pryor, T.A., Warner, H.R.: Admitting Screening at Latter-Day Saints Hospital. In Davies, D.F. (Edit.): Health Evaluation. An Entry to the Health Care System. Intercontinental Medical Book Co., New York 1973.

56. Ramcharan, S., Cutler, J.L., Feldman, R., Siegelaub, A.B., Campbell, B., Friedman, G.D., Dales, L.G., Collen, M.F.: Multiphasic Checkup Evaluation Study: 2. Disability and Chronic Disease after Seven Years of Multiphasic Checkups. Prev.Med. 2 (1973) 207-220.

57. Roberts, N.J.: The Values and Limitations of Periodic Health Examinations. J.chron.Dis. 9 (1959) 95-116.

58. Roberts, N.J., Ipsen, J., Elsom, K.O., Clark, T.W., Yanagawa, H.: Mortality among Males in Periodic Health Examination Programs. New Engl.J.Med. 28 (1969) 20-24.

59. Rosen, G.: Preventive Medicine in the United States, 1900-1975, Trends and Interpretations. N. Watson, New York 1976.

60. Sackett, D.L., Holland, W.W.: Controversy in the Detection of Disease. Lancet 1975, II: 357-359.

61. Schoen, A.V.: AMHT Program Directory, International 1972-73. 3rd Ed. Bioscience Pub., Burbank, Calif. 1973.

62. Schweitzer, S.O.: Cost Effectiveness of Early Detection of Disease. Hlth Serv.Res. 9 (1974) 22-32.

63. Sharp, C.L., Keen, H.: Presymptomatic Detection and Early Diagnosis. Pitman Med.Pub.Co., Ltd., London 1968.

64. Siegel, G.S.: Periodic Health Examinations. Abstracts from the Literature. Publ.Hlth Serv. Publ.No. 1010. U.S.Govt.Print Off., Washington, DC 1963.

65. Soghikian, K., Collen, F.B.: Acceptance of Multiphasic Screening Examinations by Patients. Bull.N.Y.Acad.Med. 45 (1969) 1366-1375.

66. Spitzer, W.D., Brown, B.P.: Unanswered Questions about the Periodic Health Examination. Ann.intern.Med. 83 (1975) 257-263.

67. Statement on Multiphasic Testing. American Medical Association, Chicago, Ill. 1972.

68. Steenwyk, J.V.: Implementing Programs for Preventive Health Care Services. Blue Cross Repts. Res. Series 2, 1969.

69. Thorner, R.M.: The Status of Activity in Automated Health Testing in the U.S.. In Automated Multiphasic Health Testing. Engineering Foundation Research Conferences. Engineering Foundation, New York 1971.

70. Thorner, R.M., Remein, Q.M.: Principles and Procedures in the Evaluation of Screening for Disease. Publ.Hlth Serv. Publ. No. 846, U.S.Govt.Print.Off., Washington, D.C. 1961.

71. Watts, M.S.: Some General Principles and Some General Guidelines. Section II. In Provisional Guidelines for Automated Multiphasic Health Testing Services. Vol. 1. 1970. National Technical Information Service (NTIS), Springfield, Va.PB 195 654.

72. Whitby, L.G.: Screening for Disease: Definitions and Criteria. Lancet 1974, II: 819-821.

73. Wilson, J.M.G., Hilleboe, H.E.: Mass Health Examinations. Public Health Paper No. 45. Geneva, W.H.O. 1971.

74. Wilson, J.M.G., Jungner, G.: Principles and Practice of Screening for Disease. Public Health Paper No. 34, Geneva, W.H.O. 1968.

75. Zucker, L.W., et al.: Cost and Cost Analysis Guidelines. Part IV. Provisional Guidelines for Automated Multiphasic Health Testing Services, Vol. 3. DHEW Publ.No. (HSM) 72-3011, 1970. U.S. Govt.Print.Off., Washington, D.C.

Periodic Health Evaluation of Individuals

P.F.L. Hall

Introduction

Multiphasic health screening centres and health maintenance clinics
are new aids to preventive care both as health protection for a
population and as health promotion for the individual (3, 4, 7, 9).
A modern health care delivery system must concern itself with the
evaluation of health as well as of disease detection. The decision-
making process for diagnostic, therapeutic and prognostic problems
has been analyzed, and there seems to be a growing feeling that
the traditional statistical-mathematical systems will not be
sufficient in the future (6). New analytical systems have been
searched for, and during recent years predictors, indicators and
health indices have been described (9). However, before details
can be presented, the difference between the decision-making
process in clinical practice (patient care) and in paraclinical
service units should be discussed.

The Model of Clinical Decision-Making

The clinical decision-making model uses as the primary information
components symptoms, signs and tests (Figure 1).

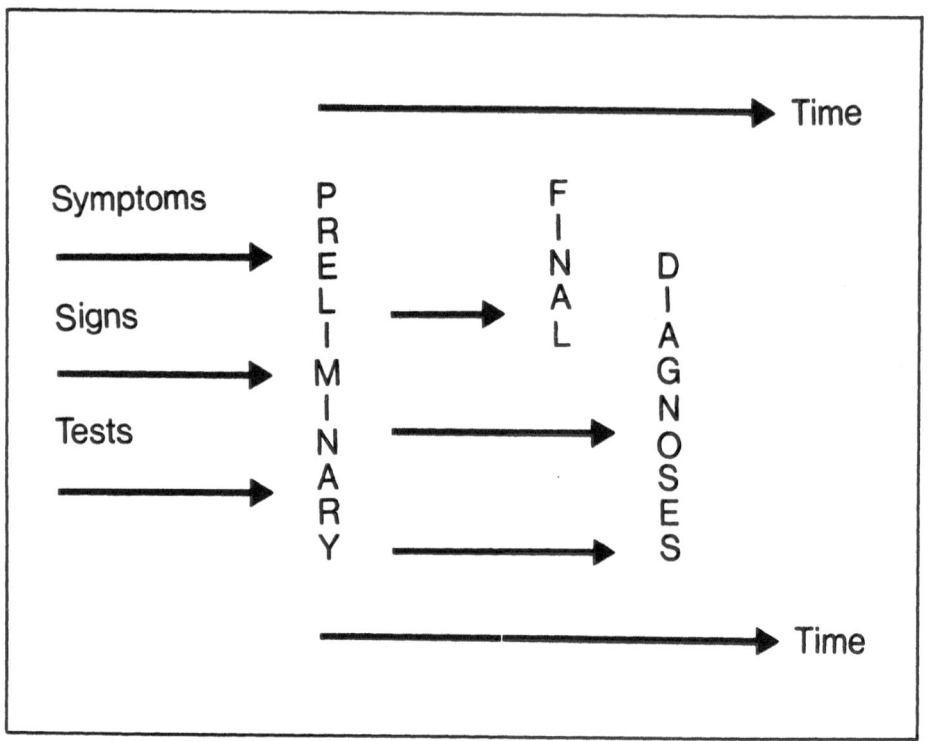

Fig. 1: Clinical decision model

The model is dynamic and the change of each bit of information
over time is vital. Trend analysis is a major part of this model.
The information accumulated from symptoms, signs and tests is
summarized in preliminary diagnoses and/or in final diagnoses.
The different diagnoses or problems have different degrees of
certainty, and one individual patient very often has more than one
problem.

Thus, in the clinical decision-making model the trend or the change
over time in symptoms, signs and tests is the criterion for
judgment. These primary information components are then summarized
into the secondary ones - the diagnoses.

In "Introduction to Medical Decision-making" Lusted (11) wrote:
"The relationship of treatment to diagnosis is that the patient's
response to treatment may be regarded as a diagnostic test whose
outcome may modify the physician's opinion about diagnosis, about
further treatment or both". The traditional mathematical-
statistical systems are difficult to apply to this dynamic
diagnostic model in which the individual is his own control.

Emlet (2) gives another example of the dynamic clinical model:
"Five days before a scheduled lunar launch one of the astronauts
was found to have a white blood count of 8,000. Neither in the
population generally nor among the astronauts as a group would
this be considered abnormal. But the astronaut in question normally
had a white blood count of 4,000. The launch was postponed; the
astronaut in question almost immediately developed an upper
respiratory infection and soon thereafter the two other crew
members developed the same problem". Please observe: At the moment
the launch was postponed, there was only a deviation from the
individual's own "normality" in one test and no diagnosis. This
description is a good example of the dynamic diagnostic model.

The Model of Paraclinical Decision-Making

Clinical information can be looked upon as the symptoms and signs
directly obtained from the patient,and the clinical decision-
making model uses these data as well as paraclinical ones in the
daily work in patient care. Paraclinical data are accumulated
from x-ray departments, chemical, physiological, bacteriological
laboratories,etc. The paraclinical decision-making model is used,
e.g., in classical medical research, in medical education and in
several laboratory routines.

The diagnosis is the primary information component in this model and the symptoms, signs and tests are secondary (Figure 2).

ONE CERTAIN DIAGNOSIS

```
┌─────────────────────────────────────────────────┐
│                                                   │
│     FREQUENCY DISTRIBUTION OF                     │
│                                                   │
│              SYMPTOMS                             │
│                                                   │
│               SIGNS                              │
│                                                   │
│               TESTS                              │
│                                                   │
│     MEAN VALUES ±  STANDARD DEVIATIONS           │
│                                                   │
└─────────────────────────────────────────────────┘
```

Fig. 2: Static, Paraclinical Model

A description of a group of patients with a certain diagnosis, e.g., in medical research, is an example of this model. The frequency distributions of signs, symptoms and tests for different age and sex groups for one diagnosis in our textbooks are other examples. The mean and two standard deviations for a laboratory test in a certain group of patients (a certain diagnosis) are a third example. The paraclinical model is static and can be said to be a descriptive non-dynamic decision model. In the patient care process the clinical and the paraclinical decision-making models are used together. There are, however, situations where the laboratory specialist has to rely upon the paraclinical model alone. The clinical hypothesis about a diagnosis may be checked by only one test at one laboratory and only once.

The paraclinical model is of great value for the overall description of different diagnoses, for medical research, for medical education and is the foundation of so-called clinical experience. It may also be stated that the paraclinical model is a simplification of a complex, complicated clinical situation. As has been stated above, neither of these models are used exclusively but they are used together. However, it is important to realize the difference between the two models when attempts are made to automate part of the decision-making process. The paraclinical model has been the traditional route for several attempts to build computer systems for decision-making. Few attempts have been made to automate the dynamic clinical model. In a recent publication other and similar aspects of the diagnostic problem have been presented (1, 14, 15, 17, 19).

Predictors, Indicators and Indices

To aid the decision-making process from the perspective of clinical practice and patient care, a new technique has been employed. The "predictive value" was first described by Vecchio (18) in 1966 and later (1974) used by Galen et al. (5) for the evaluation of laboratory data. The new technique was analyzed from a theoretical standpoint by Hall et al. (9, 10). In these papers a first attempt was made to describe the clinical and paraclinical decision-making models, and the new "values" were given the names "Predictors" and "Indicators". A predictor gives the risk of having a diagnosis with a certain positive finding. An indicator gives the chance of having no diagnosis with a certain negative finding. The index or indices are the total sum of a predictor and an indicator or several predictors and indicators.

A theory and a methodology of laboratory data evaluation (continuous variables) by indicators and predictors was described in 1975 by Sebag and Hall (13). The method - described below - is identical with the above mentioned theory and methodology. The new system, however, can be applied without modifications to binary as well as to continuous variables. The old method used for the evaluation of binary variables, e.g., no answers to anamnestic questions, is altered in a way so that all data can be analyzed in a uniform manner.

Methodology

Step 1: Database

Coded or numeric values of symptoms, signs and tests are
accumulated in the database (the medical record) together with
information about diagnosis and non-diagnosis. The method can,
however, even be used for comparisons between two different
diagnoses . In the following example the method is applied to
healthy (non-diagnosed) individuals and to diagnosed ones.

In the Multiphasic Health Center at Sophiahemmet in Stockholm the
data about diagnoses etc. are stored in a partly problem-oriented
medical record. Each problem (diagnosis) is described in free text
and the corresponding diagnosis is coded according to the
expanded version of the ICD. Data about symptoms, signs and tests
and additional information are or may be stored in the computer
medical record library "J5" (8, 12).

Step 2: Definition of intervals and distribution of non-diagnosed (healthy) and diagnosed individuals

The values, the results or the answers to a test, a sign or a
symptom are arranged in a number of intervals. E.g., the continuous
variable hemoglobine may be divided into two, three, seven or any
number of intervals. The individuals within each interval are then
divided into two groups: healthy (non-diagnosed) and diagnosed.

Example: Interval	1	2	3	4
Hemoglobine values	< 100	100-149	150-159	$\geq$ 160

The intervals for continuous variables do not have to be of equal
size (e.g., 0-19, 20-29, 40-59 units). Binary variables can
naturally only be divided into two intervals: yes/no or +/-
(Figure 3).

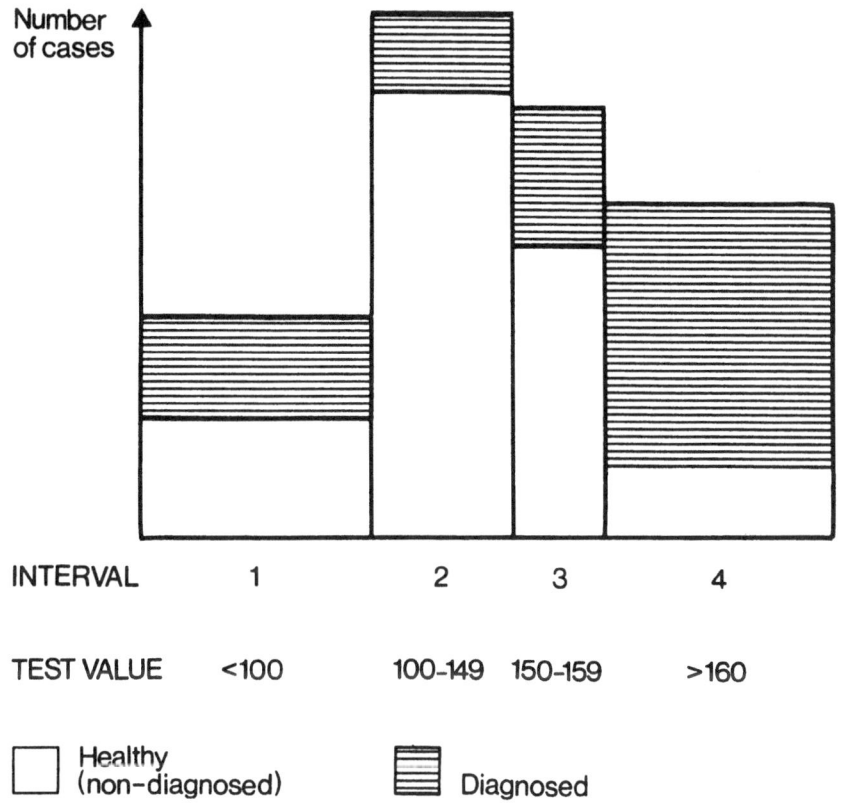

Fig. 3: Description of intervals and distribution of healthy (non-
diagnosed) and diagnosed individuals.

Step 3: Definition of maximum (optimal) health interval and
maximum health level

The optimal health interval for symptoms, signs and tests is
determined by calculating the ratio of healthy (non-diagnosed) to
all individuals for each interval. The interval with the largest
ratio is defined as the maximum health interval. The maximum health
level is defined as the border-line between the maximum health
interval and the interval with the second highest ratio.

From this level increasing as well as decreasing values may signify increasing danger or risk of diagnosis (disease) (Figure 4).

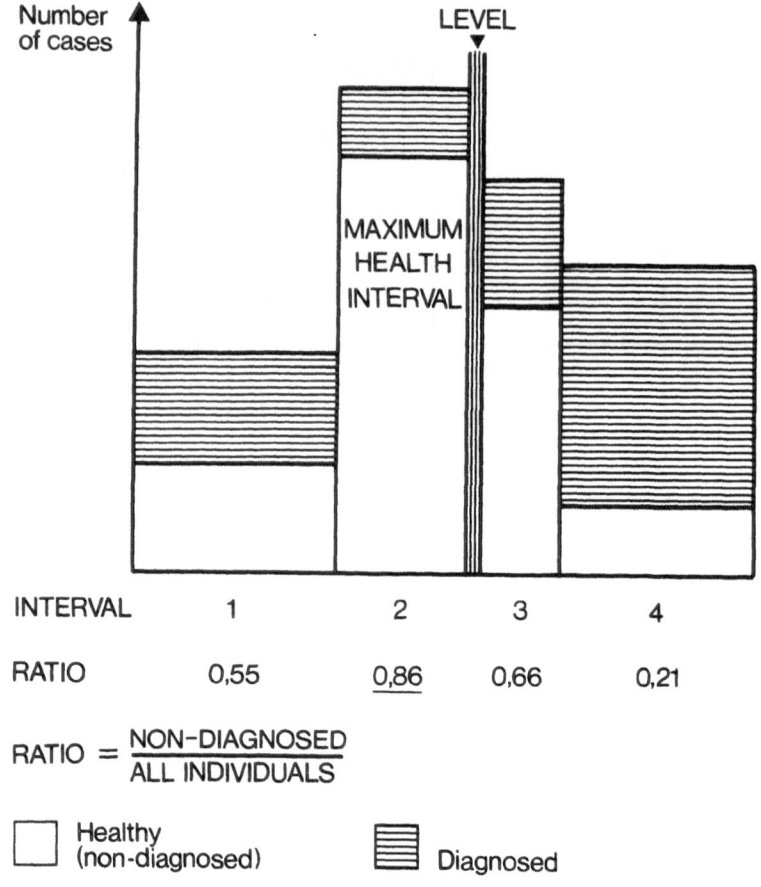

Fig. 4: Description of maximum of optimal health interval and maximum health level.

Step 4: Definition of negative and positive results of symptoms, signs and tests

Negative results of symptoms, signs and tests are defined as values falling between the midpoint of one interval and the maximum health test level. Positive results are defined as values falling between the midpoint of one interval and the extreme end of the distribution, i.e. the outermost interval at the same end of the distribution. Each interval is in this way split into two identical halves, the number of individuals in each half being identical.

The results in the distal half to the maximum health test level are defined as positive, while those in the proximal half are negative (Figures 5 and 6).

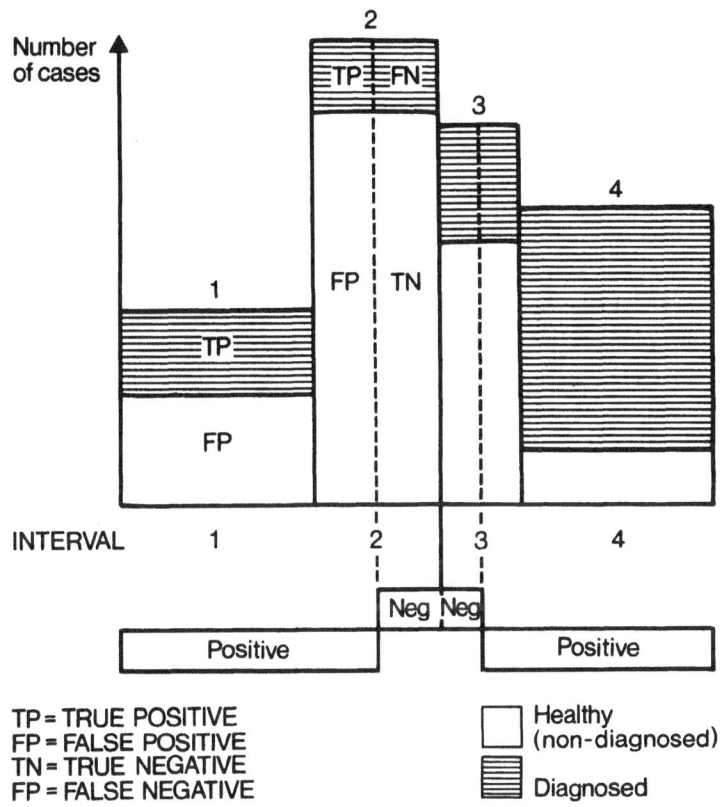

Fig. 5: Definition of negative and positive results of symptoms, signs and tests for interval 2 and 3. For definition of true and false positive, see text - step 5.

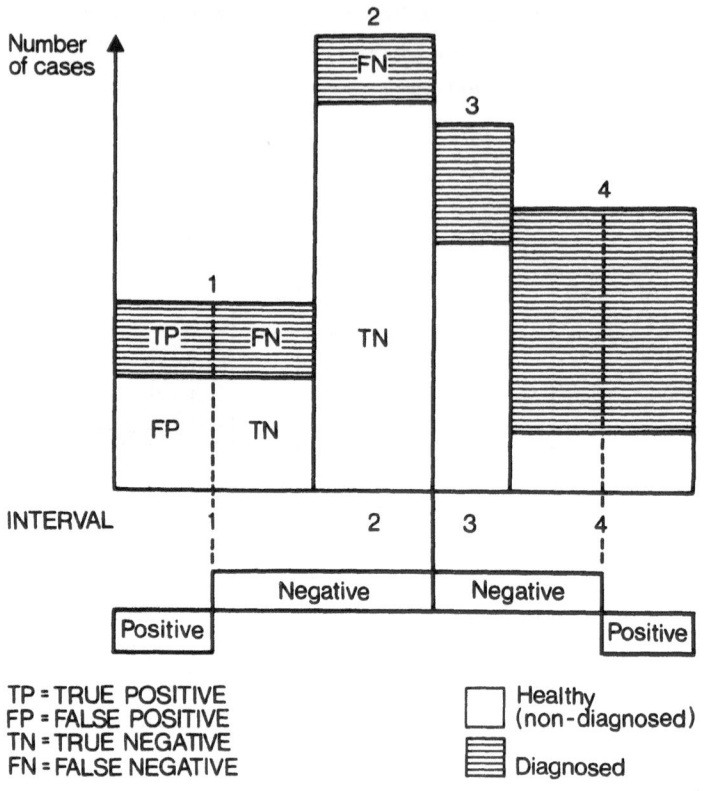

Fig. 6: Definition of negative and positive results of symptoms, signs and tests for interval 1 and 4. For definition of true and false positives see text - step 5.

Step 5: Definition of true and false positives and negatives

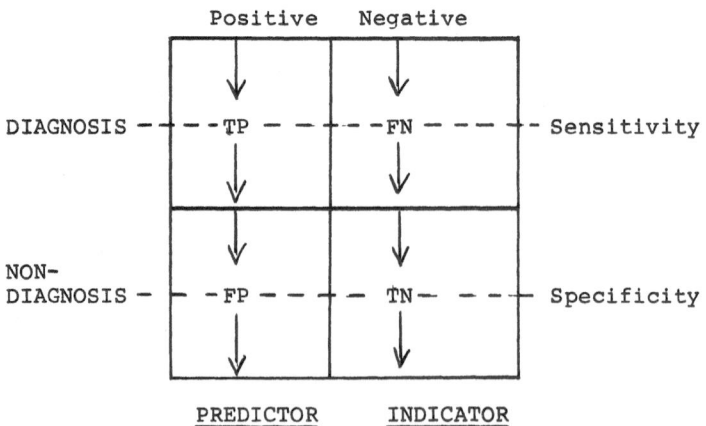

The schema above shows the fourfold table with False Negatives (FN), True Negatives (TN), False Positives (FP) and True Positives (TP). Discrete or binary results can easily be classified in this manner.

The fourfold table can be used in two different ways: One vertical and one horizontal. The horizontal way gives sensitivity and specificity which are valuable judgments in the paraclinical, static diagnostic model. Sensitivity and specificity are techniques or tools to determine the value of symptoms, signs and tests for one diagnosis. The vertical way of using the fourfold tables gives the indicator and the predictor. These two parameters can be looked upon as measures for the likelihood of health or the risk of disease (diagnosis) with one certain symptom, sign or test. The new parameters seem to be a more efficient tool in the clinical decision-making process than the old values sensitivity and specificity. The static diagnostic model with sensitivity and specificity increases our knowledge about a diagnosis, e.g., for better education of students. The dynamic diagnostic model with indicators and predictors is a tool for better patient care and for more efficient clinical decision-making.

Step 6: Definition of indicators and predictors

An indicator reflects the likelihood that a negative result indicates health (non-diagnosis), and the higher the value the greater the chance of health. The indicator is calculated as follows:

$$\text{Indicator} = \frac{TN}{TN + FN} = \frac{\text{Non-diagnosed individuals with negative findings}}{\text{All individuals with negative findings}}$$

A predictor reflects the likelihood that a positive result reflects disease (a diagnosis), and the higher the value the greater the risk of disease (diagnosis).

$$\text{Predictor} = \frac{TP}{TP + FP} = \frac{\text{Diagnosed individuals with positive findings}}{\text{All individuals with positive findings}}$$

The indicator values for an interval are highest in the maximum health interval. The indicator values may be rather low on one or both sides of the extreme ends of a distribution. The indicator has been given a positive sign and can vary from +1,0 to 0. The

opposite is true of the predictor, where the lowest values are
in the maximum health interval and the highest at the two extreme
ends of a distribution. The predictor values have been given a
negative sign and can vary from 0 to -1.0.

At this step the first analysis of the diagnostic power of the
different intervals can be made. The intervals may be rearranged,
e.g., the number of intervals may be reduced or increased. The
interval level may be changed to give a more powerful diagnostic
discrimination. Specific questions may have a very small diagnostic
significance and may be deleted or rephrased. New questions may be
added. Our experience is that this step is an important milestone
and gives valuable information about health and diagnoses for
different signs, symptoms and tests.

Step 7: Definition of a health/diagnostic index for one symptom,
        one sign or one test interval

The indicator gives the likelihood of health (non-diagnosis) and has
a positive sign. The predictor gives the risk of disease and has a
negative sign. For practical reasons, we have experimented with a
sum of the indicator and the predictor. The sum is called an index
and is defined as I+P. The index can vary from +1.0 to -1.0. When
the index is +1.0 the likelihood of health is very high, and when
it is -1.0 the risk of disease is high. The diagnostic power for an
index around 0 is low or non-existing.

Step 8: Definition of anamnestic (medical, history), chemical etc.
        indices

With coded or numeric signs, symptoms and intervals of tests it is
possible to build up an index for each one of them. Binary data
from, e.g., a self-administered questionnaire will have an index
for yes-answers and another index for no-answers (Table 1). The
diagnostic power for both kinds of answers is thus calculated. The
total diagnostic power from a questionnaire can be calculated. The
sum of all indices for yes- and no-answers given by the patient
can be said to reflect the content of the questionnaire. It has
to be remembered that in this example the method is used for the
problem health/no health (diagnoses). This diagnostic problem
should be the starting point both in health and sick care. The

Table 1: Evaluation of binary data from a self-administered questionnaire

DIAGNOSIS: BLEEDING DISORDER (von Willebrand's disease)

QUESTION 1. DO YOU SUFFER FROM A BLEEDING DISORDER?

ANSWER: NO   YES

       IND.+0,80   PRED.-0,20 | IND.+0,42   PRED.-0,58
       Indicator   Predictor

INDEX: +0,60   -0,16
       '   '   '   '
       '   '   '   '
       '   '   '   '

QUESTION 26. HAVE YOU EVER HAD A SPONTANEOUS BLEEDING?

ANSWER: NO   YES

       IND. +0,42   PRED.-0,51 | IND. 0,00   PRED.-1,00

INDEX: -0,02   -1,00
       '   '   '   '
       '   '   '   '
       '   '   '   '

QUESTION 32. DO YOU HAVE RELATIVES WHO HAVE HAD
             CORONARY AND/OR VENOUS TROMBOSIS?

ANSWER: NO   YES

       IND: 0,17   PRED.-0,83 | IND. 0,62   PRED.-0,38

INDEX: -0,66   +0,24

logical first step is to decide whether an individual is healthy
or sick. It is also a valuable tool for calculating a medical history
index in a multiphasic screening procedure. Each visit of a
patient/individual to the centre will give a new medical history
index. The change over time in this history index will immediately
give an answer to the questions: Is the patient worse, unchanged
or better?

The chemical profile, e.g., 25 different tests, can also be
summarized for each patient into a chemical index. Again the
benefit is that a change in one or several of the tests with time
will show up. A dynamic trend analysis for several tests is
possible in this way. It is important to observe that for a number
of chemical and hematological tests the diagnostic power goes in
two directions. E.g., low or high white cells may signify disease.
A chemical index must be built to take this fact into consideration.
One solution is to use one chemical index for the high values and
another for low ones. All values above the maximum health interval
are defined as high values, and low values are all values below
that interval. This method will give a guarantee that, if one test
goes upwards with time and another goes down, the change will not
cover up vital information.

An example of the use of indicators, predictors and indices is
shown in Table 1. The study was made by T. Wahlberg et al. in 1980
at the island of Åland (16). The bleeding disorder v. Willebrand's
disease was detected in this island several decades ago. However,
the study included other bleeding diseases as well. All the
individuals had to complete a detailed questionnaire with 32
questions and all blood analyses were made at the coagulation
laboratory of the Karolinska Hospital (Head: Margareta Blombäck,
M.D.). Three of the questions have been chosen as an example of how
the method can be used.

The first question: "Do you suffer from a bleeding disorder?" has a
high indicator (0.80) for a no-answer. The predictor is only -0.20.
The index of +0.60 indicates that a no-answer gives a rather great
likelihood of health. A yes-answer to the same question, however,
gives an indicator of +0.42 and a predictor of -0.58 and an index
of -0.16. The reason for this rather low diagnostic power may be
explained by the fact that several inhabitants of the island
believe that they suffer from a mild type of v. Willebrand's disease.

The second question: "Have you ever had a spotaneous bleeding?" has an index of 0.02 for a no-answer, and thus the diagnostic function is very small. A no-answer gives no information about health or disease. On the other hand, a yes-answer is a good predictor for a bleeding disorder. The risk of having a disease is very high when the predictor is -1.0 and the index is -1.0.

The third question: "Do you have relatives who have had coronary and/or venous trombosis?". A no-answer gives a low indicator and a high predictor and the index -0.66 indicates a high risk of having a bleeding disorder. The fact that individuals with, e.g., v. Wille- brand's disease have a low frequency of coronary sclerosis is demonstrated. A yes-answer on the other hand gives a likelihood of health with an index 0.24.

The medical history indices, the sum of each answer to questions, can naturally be added for each patient. E.g., if a patient had answered yes to all questions in the example, the history index would be -0.16 - 1.00 +0.24 -0.92. If all answers were no the history index would be +0.60 -0.02 -0.66 = -0.08.

Summary

A method has been described for the analysis of symptoms, signs and tests. The indicator gives the likelihood of health and the predictor gives the risk of disease. The two values can be summarized into one index for each finding. The indices for each of the findings for one patient can then be summarized into medical history indices or into a complete health index for an individual. The method will help us to monitor or follow an individual's health over an unlimited period of time.

The method is under further development and is in use for the analysis of bleeding diseases (especially v. Willebrand's disease), and a thesis will be presented by T. Wahlberg during 1980.

The problem of health and diagnosis is gaining more and more interest. The so-called minor medicine of today needs more sophisticated methods to follow not only the health of the indi- vidual but also the impact of the environment on the population (10).

References

1. Dombal, F.T.de: Medical diagnosis from a clinician's point of view.Meth. Inform. Med. 17 (1978) 28-34.

2. Emlet, H.E.: Workshop summary: Systems for evaluation of health care.In Driggs, M.F. (Edit.): Problem-directed and Medical Information Systems, p. 203 ff.
   (New York: Intercontinental Medical Book Corporation 1973).

3. Federation of Swedish County Councils (Svenska Landstingsför-bundet): Fran sjukvardspolitik till hälsopolitik (From sick-care policy to health-care policy). (Stockholm: Svenska Landstings-förbundet Publication 1974).

4. Flagle, C.D.: Automated multiphasic testing and services. Total systems analysis and design. Meth. Inform. Med. 10 (1971) 201-206.

5. Galen, R.S., Sebag, J., Gambino, S.R.: From data to information: the predictive value of laboratory tests as defined by variable referent values. Proceed. IRIA Symp. Med. Data Process., Toulouse, March 1974, Vol. 1, pp. 183-187.

6. Galen, R.S.: The normal range - a concept in transition. Arch. Path. Lab. Med. 101 (1977) 561-565.

7. Garfield, S.: The delivery of medical care. Scient. Amer. 222 (1970) 15-23.

8. Hall, P.: Computer file structure and data presentation in the Karolinska system. In Collen, M.F. (Edit.): Proceedings of an International Conference on Health Technology Systems, pp. 206-220. (San Francisco: ORSA Health Applications Section Publication 1974).

9. Hall, P., Sebag, J.: Decision-making in clinical practice and medical research: a theoretical analysis of predictors, indicators and health index. Int. J. bio-med. Comput. 5 (1974) 301-309.

10. Hall, P., Axelsson, G., Sebag, J.: Relationship between work environment and anamnestic health status. Use of predictors, indicators and indices for the evaluation of medical and environmental factors. Scand. J. Work Environ. Hlth 1 (1975) 233-242.

11. Lusted, L.B.: Introduction to Medical Decision Making, p. IX. (Springfield: C.C. Thomas 1968).

12. Mellner, C., Selander, H., Wolodarski, J.: The computerized problem-oriented medical record at Karolinska Hospital - Format and function, users' acceptance and patient attitude to questionnaire -. Meth. Inform. Med. 15 (1976) 11-20.

13. Sebag, J., Hall, P.: Decision-making in medical research and clinical practice: theory and methodology of laboratory data evaluation by predictors, indicators and indices. Meth. Inform. Med. 14 (1975) 113-117.

14. Tautu, P., Wagner, G.: The process of medical diagnosis: routes of mathematical investigations. Meth. Inform. Med. 17 (1978) 1-8.

15. Wagner, G., Tautu, P., Wolber, U.: Problems of medical diagnosis - a bibliography. Meth. Inform. Med. 17 (1978) 55-74.

16. Wahlberg, T.: Dissertation Stockholm Univ., (to be published).

17. Wardle, A., Wardle, L.: Computer aided diagnosis - a review of research. Meth. Inform. Med. 17 (1978) 15-28.

18. Vecchio, T.J.: The predictive value of a single test in unselected populations. New Engl. J. Med. 274 (1966) 1171-1173.

19. Zentgraf, R., Victor, N.: Some problems arising in the statistical treatment of diagnosis. Meth. Inform. Med. 17 (1978) 10-15.

Individual Aspects of Health - The Individual
Longitudinal Health Profile and Index

G.Z. Williams

Traditionally health assessment has been oriented to the detection
of abnormalities and disabilities or screening for disease. Almost
all health indices reported in medical and epidemiological literature
are based on morbidity or mortality statistics. The few indices
dealing with the individual assess the negative aspects of health
i.e., presence of disabilities and abnormalities *). This is not
surprising because medicine deals with disease and the profession
and society generally consider people either sick or healthy. Only
recently have at-risk states of body functions been recognized.
Unfortunately, even today the term "health" is used to mean
"medical"; and this confusion is perpetrated by the professional and
governmental designations "delivery of health care", "health care
facilities" and "health maintenance organizations", all referring
to care of the sick.

However, there are people who are healthy in a positive sense; not
merely in terms of the absence of recognizable disease, but their
chemical, physiological and psychological characteristics and
functions are optimal; they are active, vital and robust, physically
and mentally.

Our initial studies at the National Institutes of Health (1960-1970)
demonstrated, not surprisingly, that healthy people are quite
individual in their biochemical and hematological attributes (4).

---

*) These studies involved the important contributions and
   collaboration of my associates: Drs. E.K. Harris, E. Cotlove and
   Dr. D.S. Young at the National Institutes of Health and Drs. G.M.
   Widdowson, A. Seifert, C.H. Mielke, J. Penton, Mr. B. Cooil and
   Ms. M. Harnly at the Institute of Health Research.
   Supported in part by a grant from the National Institute of
   General Medical Sciences, N.I.H., Bethesda, MD, USA.

We also demonstrated that to characterize and record each person's individuality requires very precise measurement methods to minimize analytical bias or variation and permit reliable comparison of results on the same individual over long intervals if subtle changes are to be identified.

Our continuing longitudinal studies were designed to use each person as his own control. His reference base included a series of 10-12 weekly measurements for each analyte to establish his average values and ranges of variation. We found that each person is quite different from any other person in patterns of serum chemistry and hematology. Measurements of the intra-individual variation of a set of measurements of each chemical constituent revealed that the range of variation in a person is much smaller in span than the range of variation of the same measurement for a population of defined healthy people.(4). This is illustrated in Figure 1 for serum cholesterol.

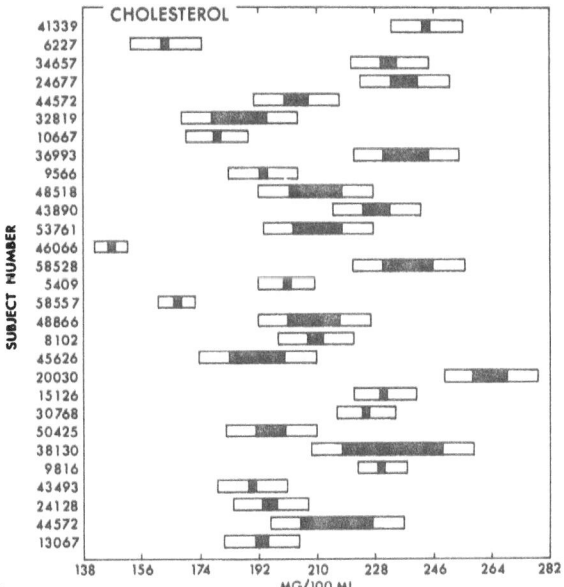

Fig. 1: Individual range of variation of serum cholesterol for each of 29 healthy people. Each bar represents the 12 weekly values. The open ends represent the estimated analytical component of variation (2) and the central solid black portion represents the estimated biological component for each person. Note the difference in level of values among the individuals and the differences in magnitude of intra-personal variations.

The same individually unique range of variation was found for all
chemical and hematological constituents. We also found that
individual variation is much the same for most constituents measured
over intervals of weeks, months or years. The ranges of variation
for urea nitrogen, uric acid, total protein, hemoglobin,
erythrocytes, hematocrit, and mean corpuscular volume for 10 and
5 weeks, 12 months and 5 and 7 years are illustrated in Figures 2a
and 2b.

```
TOTAL PROT   ( 6.2)                                                              ( 8.0)
UP 0  (10)   L...................A................H                                         6.2, 6.8/ 6.5+-  0.18
UP 1  ( 5)   ...A..............H                                                            6.0, 6.5/ 6.3+-  0.27
UP 2  ( 3)       L..........A.......H                                                       6.3, 6.7/ 6.5+-  0.18
UP 3  ( 3)                 L...A.H                                                          6.6, 6.7/ 6.7+-  0.07
UP 4  ( 5)   * RESULT OUT OF SCALE                                                          5.3, 5.8/ 5.6+-  0.24


URIC ACID    ( 2.0)                                                              ( 9.0)
UP 0  (10)             L...........A.............H                                          3.6, 5.8/ 4.6+-  0.69
UP 1  ( 3)         L........A..........H                                                    3.4, 4.9/ 4.1+-  0.78
UP 2  ( 3)              L.......A........H                                                  4.1, 5.2/ 4.7+-  0.55
UP 3  ( 3)          L....A...H                                                              3.7, 4.4/ 4.1+-  0.36
UP 4  ( 3)              L..A...H                                                            4.1, 4.8/ 4.4+-  0.34


UREA NITRO   ( 7.0)                                                              ( 27.0)
UP 0  (10)               L..................A...............H                               13.0, 21.1/ 17.8+-  2.30
UP 1  ( 3)               L........A..........H                                              14.0, 18.4/ 16.1+-  2.04
UP 2  ( 3)                       L......A......H                                            17.3, 20.3/ 18.6+-  1.50
UP 3  ( 3)                       L..........A...............H                               16.4, 21.7/ 18.4+-  2.90
UP 4  ( 3)               L..............A.........H                                         12.7, 18.9/ 16.5+-  3.35
```

Fig. 2a: Longitudinal "profile" of serum total protein, uric
          acid and urea nitrogen of one individual over a period
          of 5 years. The lower and upper limits of the 3 scales
          are designated in parentheses at the ends of the top
          line for each analyte. The baseline values - UP O
          (10) for 10 weeks determine the position and length
          of the bar L...A...H... The right hand column lists
          the lowest, highest and average values and the
          standard deviation for each consecutive annual set.
          Comparison of ranges from year to year reveals the
          variation for periods of 12 months and for the
          5 years.

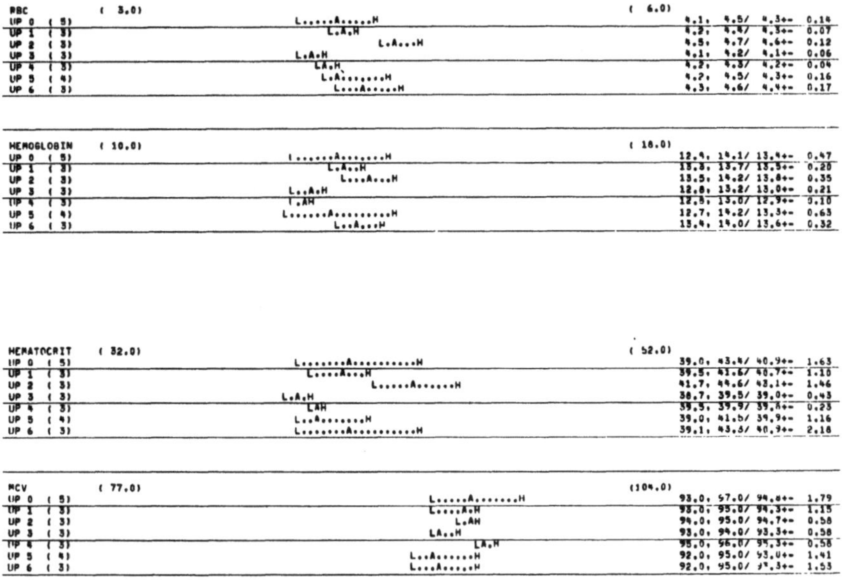

```
RBC      ( 3.0)                                            ( 6.0)
UP 0  ( 5)              L......A.....H                              4.1, 4.5/ 4.3+- 0.14
UP 1  ( 3)                  L.A.H                                   4.2, 4.6/ 4.3+- 0.07
UP 2  ( 5)                        L.A...H                           4.5, 4.7/ 4.6+- 0.12
UP 3  ( 3)             L.A..H                                       4.1, 4.2/ 4.1+- 0.06
UP 4  ( 3)                 LA.H                                     4.2, 4.3/ 4.2+- 0.04
UP 5  ( 4)                 L.A.....H                                4.2, 4.5/ 4.3+- 0.16
UP 6  ( 3)                  L...A....H                              4.3, 4.6/ 4.4+- 0.17


HEMOGLOBIN  ( 10.0)                                        ( 18.0)
UP 0  ( 5)          I......A......H                               12.4, 14.1/ 13.4+- 0.47
UP 1  ( 3)                 L.A..H                                 13.3, 13.7/ 13.5+- 0.20
UP 2  ( 3)                  L...A...H                             13.5, 14.2/ 13.8+- 0.35
UP 3  ( 3)            L..A.H                                      12.8, 13.2/ 13.0+- 0.21
UP 4  ( 3)            I.AH                                        12.6, 13.0/ 12.9+- 0.10
UP 5  ( 4)         L......A.........H                             12.7, 14.2/ 13.3+- 0.63
UP 6  ( 3)                L..A..H                                 13.4, 14.0/ 13.6+- 0.32


HEMATOCRIT  ( 32.0)                                        ( 52.0)
UP 0  ( 5)           L.......A..........H                         39.0, 43.4/ 40.9+- 1.63
UP 1  ( 3)           L....A...H                                   39.5, 41.6/ 40.7+- 1.10
UP 2  ( 3)                   L......A......H                      41.7, 44.6/ 43.1+- 1.46
UP 3  ( 3)        L.A.H                                           38.7, 39.6/ 39.0+- 0.43
UP 4  ( 3)              LAH                                       39.5, 39.9/ 39.7+- 0.23
UP 5  ( 4)           L..A.....H                                   39.0, 41.6/ 39.9+- 1.16
UP 6  ( 3)           L.......A..........H                         39.1, 43.6/ 40.9+- 2.18


MCV      ( 77.0)                                          (104.0)
UP 0  ( 5)                     L......A......H                    93.0, 97.0/ 94.4+- 1.79
UP 1  ( 3)                     L....A.H                           93.0, 95.0/ 94.3+- 1.15
UP 2  ( 3)                       L.AH                             94.0, 95.0/ 94.7+- 0.58
UP 3  ( 3)                    LA..H                               93.0, 94.0/ 93.3+- 0.58
UP 4  ( 3)                       LA.H                             95.0, 96.0/ 95.3+- 0.58
UP 5  ( 4)                  L..A.....H                            92.0, 95.0/ 93.0+- 1.41
UP 6  ( 3)                  L....A....H                           92.0, 95.0/ 93.3+- 1.53
```

Fig. 2b: Longitudinal bar chart of a person's profile of
         hematological constituents for 6 years. Note the
         remarkably narrow ranges of variation and
         consistency over the long term.

These observations support the concept that the individual pattern
of chemical and physiological functions for a given person remains
quite stable over time as long as the person remains healthy and the
assumption that changes in average levels and increasing ranges of
variation (in comparison to his former pattern) indicate either
the deterioration of that function portending development of an
abnormality, or an improving adaptation to environment (change of
lifestyle, etc.). This method of establishing a prior record of
time-series sets of averages and ranges for each person should be
a powerful and sensitive tool for detecting change.

Our studies of 2,200 healthy people in San Francisco were designed
to test this concept. We accepted participants classified as healthy
by a working definition including a negative physical examination,
absence of known disease, and no recognizable abnormalities in a
battery of laboratory tests. Subjects under a physician's care for
any purpose or taking any therapeutic medication were excluded.
These people have been followed from three to eight years with
annual assessments. Each examination included a comprehensive health,
lifestyle and stress questionnaire, several physiological measurements (weight, resting heart rate and resting blood pressure) and
three to five sets of weekly blood analyses. Blood serum and cellular
assays were performed with rigid quality control in an automated
instrumental system transmitting assay signals directly to our
research computer. Coded questionnaire responses obtained at the
same time as the blood specimens were also entered into each
person's computer files via punched cards. Permanent mass storage
includes over 1,000,000 data items on these 2,200 subjects.

Using appropriate statistical and correlation programs and with the
collaboration of Dr. Harris (Chief, Laboratory of Applied Studies,
Division of Computer Research and Technology, National Institutes
of Health, Bethesda, MD) we have estimated the intraindividual
variation and means of each attribute for each person, both for
the initial 5 week reference period and for the annual update
periods, Table 1.

Table 1: Average Intra-Individual Range of Variation
for 95 Healthy Subjects. Variance Expressed
as Coefficient of Variation:
Comparison of Initial Base-Line Set of 5
Weekly Samples with all Samples Collected
Annually for 3 - 5 Years.

Constituent	Initial 5 Weekly		All Samples	
	Mean	CV%	Mean	CV%
Calcium	4.7	3	4.7	3
Magnesium	1.65	8	1.65	7
Urea Nitrogen	16.2	14	16.5	27
Glucose	88	9	88	9
Total Protein	7.1	3	7.0	4
Cholesterol	206	8	210	9
Triglycerides	107	28	106	32
Uric Acid	5.4	9	5.5	10
Phosphate	3.3	8	3.3	10
Creatinine	1.0	8	1.0	7
Aspartate Transaminase	15.6	20	14.2	28
Lactate Dehydrogenase	64	11	62	13
Alkaline Phosphatase	44	10	42	14
Creatine Kinase	33	33	36	55
Gamma Glutamyl Transferase	19	33	21	66
Thyroxin (T4)	4.9	13	4.9	12
Leukocytes	5.4	11	5.3	12
Erythrocytes	4.6	3	4.6	3
Hemoglobin	14.2	3	14.1	3
Hematocrit	42	1	42	2
Mean Cell Volume	92	0.5	91	0.6
Platelets	188	8	210	15

The average ranges of intra-individual variation which were
determined by analysis of variance are listed for a group of 95
healthy subjects, for their initial reference set of 5 or 10 weekly
results and for their entire series of results over a 3 - 5 year
period. The average range of variation is expressed as coefficient
of variation. Comparison of the two sets demonstrates that for all
blood constituents except urea nitrogen, triglycerides, aspartate
amino transferase, creatine kinase, gamma glutamyl transferase and
platelets the ranges of variation for 5 or 10 weeks are identical
or very similar to the 3 - 5 year range.

This observation is also apparent in the individual chronological
bar graphs. The bar graph of ranges of variation for several serum
chemicals in one subject for several years is reproduced in Figure 3.

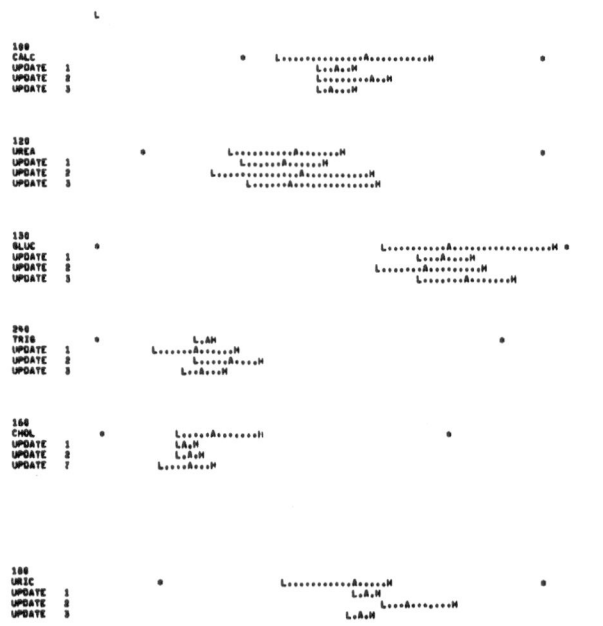

Fig. 3: Typical bar graph of an individual profile of 6
of the 16 serum chemical constituents measured
in annual sets of 5 or 3 weekly results for 4 years.

This is a typical pattern indicating homeostatic stability we find characteristic in a healthy person.

All results for the complete battery of laboratory tests for each update period are displayed in this convenient format. Visual review permits immediate recognition of deviations from the person's reference base (update 0) or prior results and facilitates identification of associations of 2 or more aberrations in his laboratory test profile. We have discovered gradual and persistent changes in mean values and ranges of variation over periods of several years. An example of a deviation is indicated in Figure 4.

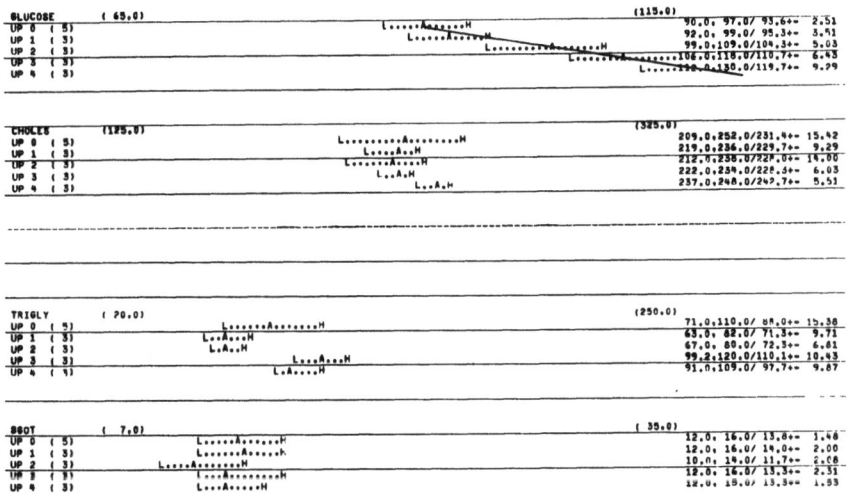

Fig.4: Portion of an individual's chemical profile showing a gradual but persistent rise in serum glucose over the 5 year period. Nevertheless, all values are within "normal limits".

There is a small but persistent increase of the mean value of glucose in update periods of 1, 2, 3, 4. The persistent and unidirectional change indicates a high probability that it will continue unless successful intervention is initiated. Note that these increases leave all values well within the limits of values generally accepted as normal. Thus our findings indicate that this time-series method of assessment for an individual is very sensitive for detecting small but persistent changes well within the limits of conventionally accepted "normality" but outside the person's own reference base, and these changes may represent early evidence of developing abnormality.

To test our assumption that such changes are significant indicators and possibly predictive, it is necessary to search for correlation of each change with concomitant alteration in general health or with time-related events in the person's life such as stress or modification of lifestyle. Each person must be monitored for sufficient years to determine the ultimate outcome of the observed change.

For this purpose we developed a Health Practice Index which is derived by a computer program from a person's questionnaire responses. The questionnaire includes categories of activity, attitude and subjective self-satisfaction, psychological energy, physical activity, alcohol and tobacco use, nutritional habits and an overall composite score. Each is appraised on a percentile scale (Figure 5) which is based on the distribution of responses of 1,670 healthy subjects.

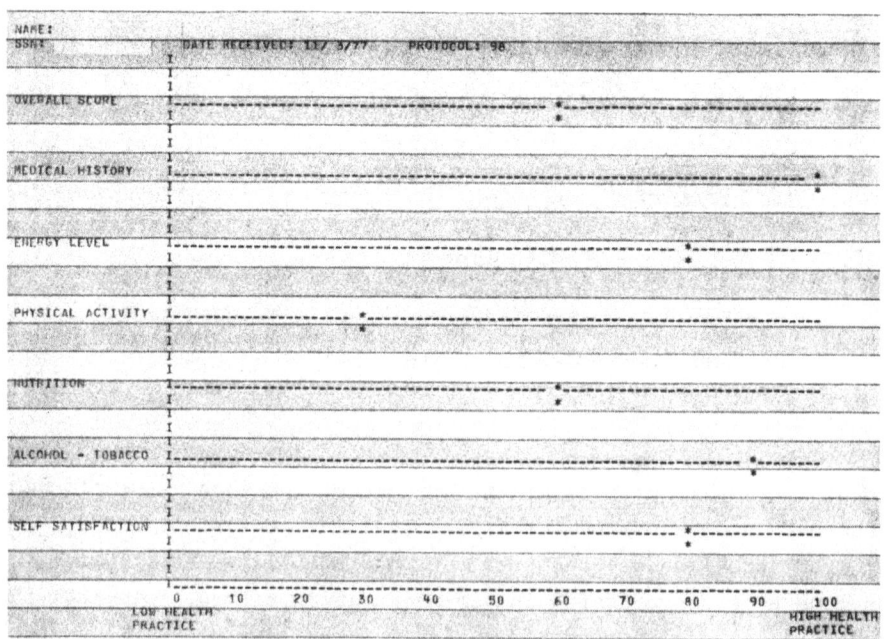

Fig. 5: Typical individual Health Practice Index chart. The double asterisks relate this person's level of health practices and reactions to the bottom scale.

As life events and exposure to stress occur and habits are altered from year to year, the person's Health Practice Index scores are expected to change and reveal an improvement or deterioration in one or more of the categories and the composite scale. This quantified assessment of "positive health" permits application of appropriate analytical programs to determine correlation of events and modifications in lifestyle with changes in profiles of laboratory measurements. A conceptual diagram of this approach and its future potential development, as more sophisticated methods become available, is suggested in Figure 6.

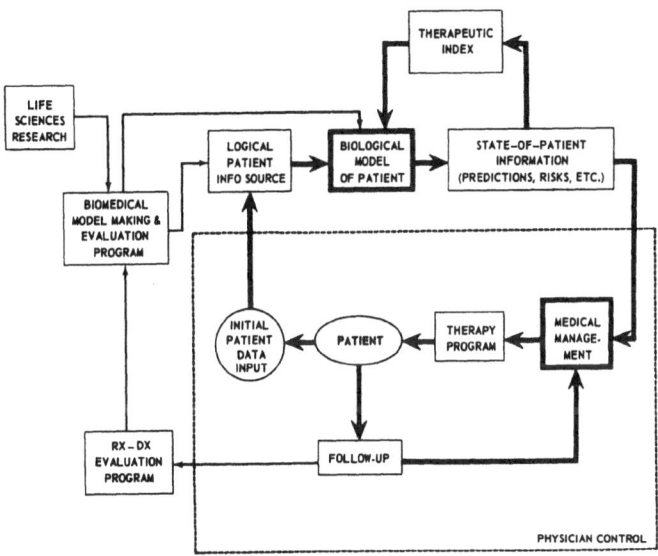

Fig. 6: Conceptual diagram of functional components and input sources for a profile model-building program

This longitudinal study of the individual avoids the problem of obscuring small but significant changes in the person by the averaging effects of analyzing group data. On the other hand, by accumulating classes of individuals who manifest similar qualitative changes and similar correlations with life events and style, we may be able to gain valuable insight into the procedures required to maintain optimum health in the individual as a basis for rational preventive medicine.

Two examples will illustrate this potential.

The serum enzyme gamma glutamyl transferase appears to reflect
liver function in relation to alcohol consumption as well as other
types of injuries. We estimated amounts of alcohol consumption for
each person as the number of drinks per week and correlated this
factor with the individual serum levels of GGT over time.
Figure 7 displays the relation of the number of drinks per week to

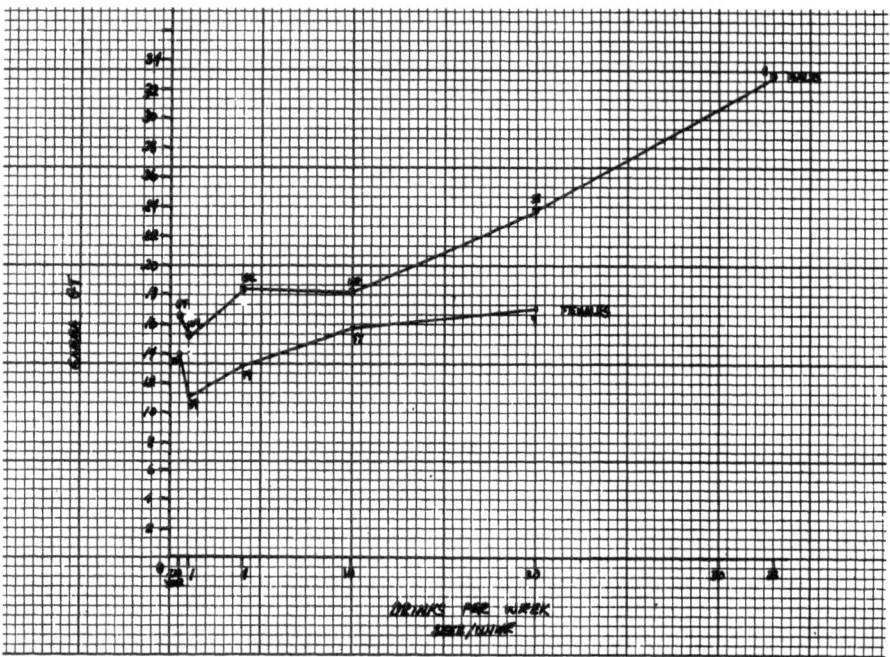

Fig. 7: Relation of moderate alcohol use to levels of serum
        gamma glutamyl transferase. The number of individuals
        reporting the different amounts of beer or wine
        consumption are indicated at the respective points
        on the curves. Similar but sharper rises were found
        for use of hard liquor.

the average level of serum GGT for a group of healthy people. The
association is striking in spite of the quantitative inadequacy
of estimating alcohol intake.

Ms. E.E. had significant increases in aspartate aminotransferase, lactate dehydrogenase and creatine kinase in her first annual update sample compared to her reference baseline values, but not high enough to be diagnostic of acute liver or muscle damage. Increases continued the second and third week (Figure 8), but all

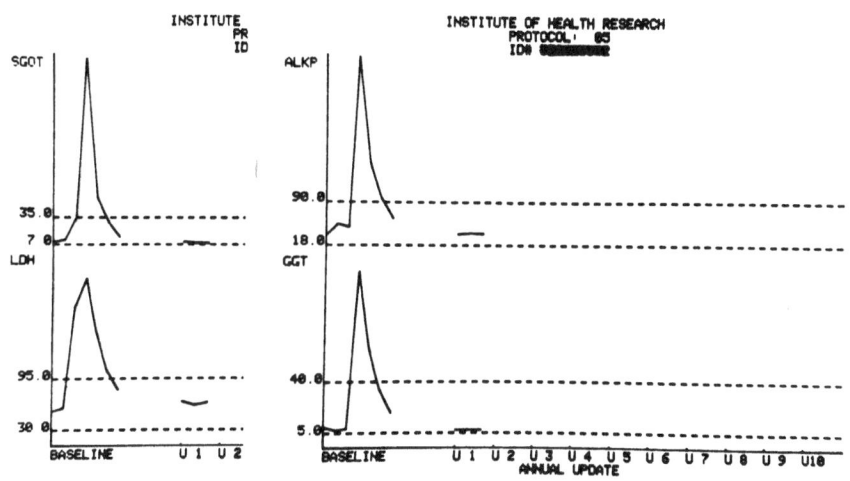

Fig. 8: Serum values of liver enzymes during a 7 week period. Note that except for LDH the first 3 weekly values, although rising, were within "normal" limits. These alerted us to continue monitoring this person until values returned almost to her previous base-line. The next annual update (U1) values are consistent with her original levels.

values declined to near her previous normal range by the 6th week. Search of her update questionnaire data revealed a time-related period of unusual fatigue, langour, slight backache and one day of mild diarrhea and headache. The evidence suggests a transient, subclinical viral hepatitis. We found six similar cases in a period of three months. However, without records of each person's previous healthy range of variation these deviations could not have been recognized.

These examples clearly indicate the potential of the individual
health profile for monitoring a person's health and tailoring
management to his needs for maintaining optimum fitness.

Basic to primary health maintenance and prevention of degenerative
disease is the detection of early changes in body chemistry,
physiology and behavioral reactions and the identification of risk
states which may be reversed or at least arrested by appropriate
intervention.

Our studies and collaborative findings of other investigators will
provide a refined definition of "normal" reference value limits
for use in both health monitoring and medical care (1,2,3,5,6).

References

(1) Belloc, N.B., Breslow, L., Hochstim, J.: Measurement of
    Physical Health in a General Population Survey.
    Amer.J.Epidemiol. 93 (1971) 328-336.

(2) Siest, G., Schiele, F., Galteau, M.-M., Panek, E., Steinmetz, J.,
    Fagnani, F., Gueguen, R.: Aspartate Aminotransferase and
    Alanine Aminotransferase Activities in Plasma: Statistical
    Distributions, Individual Variations, and Reference Values.
    Clin.Chem. 21 (1975) 1077-1087.

(3) Statland, B.E., Winkel, P.: Variations of Cholesterol and
    Total Lipid Concentrations in Sera of Healthy Young Men.
    Amer.J.clin.Path. 66 (1976) 935-943.

(4) Williams, G.Z., Young, D.S., Stein, M.R., Cotlove, E.:
    Biological and Analytic Components of Variation in Long-term
    Studies of Serum Constituents in Normal Subjects. I. Objectives,
    Subject Selection, Laboratory Procedures, and Estimation of
    Analytic Deviation. Clin.Chem. 16 (1970) 1016-1021.

(5) Yasaka, T.: Health Control Data-base System and Subject-specific
    Normal Range. Med.Inform. 1 (1976) 105-132.

(6) Young, D.S., Harris, E.K., Cotlove, E.: Biological and Analytic
    Components of Variation in Long-term Studies of Serum
    Constituents in Normal Subjects. IV. Results of a Study
    Designed to Eliminate Long-term Analytic Deviations.
    Clin.Chem. 17 (1971) 403-410.

Rural Community Health Information Acquisition

Roger A. Côté

In most countries the delivery of health care to rural communities
has improved over the last decade. Governments have given incentives
to physicians to settle in rural communities, and in some countries
it has become mandatory for young physicians to serve in rural areas
at the start of their career.

In Canada, especially in Quebec, socialization of medicine has
brought government-sponsored intervention in the rural areas. One
step in the right direction has been the investment by government in
the building of community health clinics called "CLSC" or "centre
local de santé communautaire". This is in essence a local community
health center. These vary in size and type of service depending on
the availability of social workers, nurses and physicians.

Because the provincial government is now paying for all health
services, it is beginning to demand more information from all health
care providers, whether institution, health clinic or solo
practitioner. Medical records must be kept by all and inspection of
these records is being accomplished by teams of physicians under the
supervision of the Professional Corporation of Physicians of Quebec.

Up to the present health care information contained in rural health
records has been untapped because it is fragmentary, uncoded and
mostly unusable. Many records in physicians offices contain only a
few handwritten, frequently scribbled notes. This must change if
rural health care information is to be integrated with better
organized data from hospitals, institutes and clinics.

Hospitals in the past decades were obliged to code mortality data
and then morbidity data for general statistical purposes. For this,
the International Classification of Diseases (ICD) (6,7) or one of
its many derivatives (2,4,10) was the recommended tool. This tool
was not in use in rural areas because of the lack of trained
personnel, medical initiative or demonstrated need.

Advanced medical and computer technology, coupled with the social awareness of quality & cost of care, has clearly demonstrated that a general classification of diseases, originally designed for mortality statistics, is incapable of managing individual patient care data for both medical audit (3) and disease costing.

The trend in sophisticated centers is to use not a general classification, but a more specific integrated nomenclature of signs, symptoms, causes, diseases and procedures. If this new approach can give us a better health care management tool, have we now left the less sophisticated rural health care further behind? Will all rural health care data be lost forever? Will there be no input from and no feedback to the rural community?

This particular problem has been in the forefront of many discussions within the Committee on Nomenclature and Classification of Disease that is responsible for the continuing development of the Systematized Nomenclature of Medicine (SNOMED) (9). We now feel that the problem can be solved and the answers will permit the modernized acquisition of rural health care data.

First, it is believed that rural health care information should consist of a core of common basic data compatible with that of urban centers, and that all health record information, although less complete or specific, should be compatible with that obtained from more sophisticated centers.

In a second phase, the cooperation of rural health care providers should be sought to obtain better information. These may be the nurse, nurse-practitioner, physician, rural health clinic or hospital. All of these providers should be made aware of the fact that not only do they frequently refer patients to a regional hospital but there is also a simultaneous transfer of information which must be compatible to ensure the quality of care. One must then examine closely the data acquisition methods available to rural health care personnel. The oldest and still most common is the handwritten or typewritten natural language. It is most frequently uncoded. Important diseases or final diagnoses may be coded at the source of the document or by regional personnel. The most desirable situation would be the development of automatic computer-assisted encoding of the natural medical language data, a technique still in its infancy.

If rural data acquisition is to be,enhanced the choice of the
method will depend on many factors:

1) the type of data needed,
2) the use to be made of the data,
3) the availability of personnel,
4) the qualifications of that personnel,
5) the type of equipment to be used,
6) the availability of access to a computer,
7) the amount and availability of funds for this function.

The methods may vary from area to area, but the use of the information,
from the basic data set to the health information per se should
be standardized.

The health information can be easily coded, either where the
information is generated, or at the regional level if the information
is collected, prepared and presented in a standard format. Coding
can be done with a personal or regional code, which is the least
desirable option. One could use a classification with its drawbacks.
A nomenclature would be the most specific, but its size and need
for trained personnel create a definite disadvantage, unless, of
course, a small subset of the nomenclature can be developed to fit
the need of the rural health community. This should contain simple
signs, symptoms and diagnoses. Furthermore, it should contain a small
list of the procedures done in that particular community.

This brings us to the concept of the microglossary. SNOMED, for
example, is the most complete medical nomenclature recently
developed for health information management (1). The first edition
consisted of 6 volumes,each one representing a different axis. There
were approximately 50,000 entries covering Topography, Morphology,
Etiology, Function, Disease and Procedure. The second edition in
two volumes has a few thousand additional terms plus a new axis
called Occupation (5). Because this nomenclature differs
philosophically from the usual one axis classification, it does take
additional training for the personnel. Having considered all these
factors,we now are developing subsets (8) of SNOMED called
microglossaries. They have been found most useful for specialty
groups and for ambulatory care. Such an approach could prove of
immense value to rural health communities for the integration of
their data. This microglossary would be compatible with SNOMED and,
by using the implosion/explosion technique, data could be source-

coded by relatively untrained personnel.

To explain this concept,let us take the microglossary developed for ambulatory care. A first draft was made at the University Medical Center at Sherbrooke and then further developed by Doctor David Shires at Halifax, Nova Scotia for the Maritime Ambulatory Record System (MARS project). This was later refined by Dr. Ronald Beckett of the Hartford Hospital, Hartford, Conn. for testing in the Hartford area hospitals. It consists mainly of about 50 typewritten pages of common signs, symptoms, diseases, and procedures divided into sections. One section is general and the others are system-oriented.

Basically, a simple alphanumeric code is given to a simple or complex entity. On the right is placed the more complex single or multiple axis SNOMED code. With this simple method, if the source of the data is identified as coming from an ambulatory care facility, the computer program would automatically explode the simple code to its more complex SNOMED code and store the data accordingly. This data is now compatible with the more sophisticated hospital data.

The following two tables show the simplicity of the method once the microglossary is assembled.

Table 1: Ambulatory Care Microglossary -
         General Section

Simple code	Term	SNOMED Explosion
G-01	Ache	F-82960
G-04	Pain and tenderness abdominal	T-Y4100 - F-82750
G-23	Tired/Fatigue/Tiredness	F-01610
G-28	Smoking, excessive	F-02850

Table 2: Ambulatory Care Microglossary -
Genito-Urinary System

Simple code	Term	SNOMED Explosion
U-3	Bleeding/urethra Hemorrhage/urethra	T-75000 - M-37000
U-6	Burning on urination	T-74000 - F-66240
U-15	Cancer of cervix	T-83000 - M-80003
U-34	Painful periods/ menstrual cramps/ dysmenorrhea	F-30200

It is therefore believed that rural health care data should be
collected in a simple manner at the source and coded easily using a
specially developed subset of SNOMED. This method will ensure the
compatibility of the data with that coming from more sophisticated
centers. Furthermore, the proper use and management of this data
will eventually permit rural medical audit and disease costing
which will further generate the utilization statistics
necessary for better health care management of the rural community.

References

1. Côté, R.A., Robboy, S.: Progress in Medical Information Management
   - Systematized Nomenclature of Medicine (SNOMED). JAMA, vol 243,
   no. 8, (1980) pp. 756 - 762.

2. Eighth Revision International Classification of Diseases,
   Adapted for Use in the United States. Public Health Service
   publication no. 1963, undated.

3. Gantner, G.E.: SNOMED Enhancement of MAN/MACHINE Medical Audits.
   Read before the American Society for Quality Control, 32nd
   Annual Technical Conference, Chicago, May 8-10, 1978 (Trans-
   actions, pp. 445-450).

4. Hospital Adaptation of ICDA (H-ICDA), ed 1. Ann Arbor, Mich, 1968, and ed 2, September 1973.

5. International Standard Classification of Occupations, revised edition. Geneva, International Labour Office, 1968.

6. Manual of the International Statistical Classification of Diseases, Injuries, and Causes of Death, ed 8. Geneva, World Health Organization, 1969.

7. Manual of the International Statistical Classification of Diseases, Injuries, and Causes of Death: Ninth Revision of the International Classification of Diseases, Geneva, World Health Organization, 1977.

8. Systematized Nomenclature of Dermatology (SNODERM), Chicago, American Academy of Dermatology, 1978.

9. Systematized Nomenclature of Medicine (SNOMED), ed 2, Skokie, I11., College of American Pathologists, 1979.

10. The International Classification of Diseases, Ninth Revision, Clinical Modification (ICD-9CM). Ann Arbor, Mich, Commission on Professional and Hospital Activities, 1978.

Information Systems for Rural Health:
Problems and Potential Benefits

D.A.B. Lindberg

Computer-based medical information systems can serve patients
directly and personally in only a very limited number of ways. These
include, for example, obtaining the interrogative patient history;
interpretation of physiological signals such as electrocardiogram
spirogram, electromyogram; and monitoring of intensive care by
sampling of patient measurements and treatment interventions.

In contrast, computers can render substantial services to persons
and to populations when they function as medical information
systems (MIS's). Rural populations are especially in need of such
services because of the sparcity of health professionals and
facilities available to them. The practicality and importance of
MIS's has been demonstrated both in rural and metropolitan settings
(1, 6). Yet this technology is far from widely disseminated, and its
development is still incomplete. Before examining problems that
are peculiar to the rural situation, it may be worthwhile to make
a formal characterization of MIS's, and to consider generally the
barriers to diffusion of MIS technology per se. This material is
presented more fully in a forthcoming book (4).

Characterization of Medical Information Systems

All MIS's contain at least the following minimal essential data:
patient identification; hospital or ambulatory care location;
demographic information; past hospitalizations; diagnoses; linkage
information relating to records obtained at various places and
times; and time/date qualifiers. In addition, MIS's have included
various combinations of the many optional data elements. These
include: billing information; physician(s) identification; invariant
physiological information; elements of health status provided by

the patient; results of measurements or observations performed upon the patient; and interpretive information. In order to assess the extent to which MIS's have been successful and in order to compare and contrast the various systems, one may properly look at each as necessarily having at least one attribute or value for each of the following dimensions:

1. Data Elements Collected (essential and optional, as noted above);

2. Medical Service Areas (e.g. clinical laboratory, intensive care, mental health, etc.);

3. Functions Performed (e.g. physician assistance functions, analysis for quality of care, analysis for refining medical knowledge, etc.);

4. Patient Population (e.g. worried well, chronically ill, etc.);

5. Uses of the Output of the System (e.g. by patient's physician, consultant, research investigator, health administrator);

6. Financial Support of System Costs.

Barriers to Diffusion of MIS Technology

It is clear that the MIS technology is still developmental. That is, its feasibility has been shown, but a full understanding of its best uses and ultimate medical benefits are not yet at hand. This situation is reflected in the U.S. in the relatively large numbers of computing systems in use in hospitals for administrative purposes, the much smaller number of medical applications of MIS's and the handful of MIS's which actually explore new medical functions and services (4).

A study of the reports by MIS developers in the U.S. suggests that three separate kinds of problems were encountered in creation and implementation of MIS's. These were: technical problems (e.g. poor terminals, no back-up computer, unreliable telephone lines, complex programming systems, etc.); social/behavioral problems (e.g. clinics' resistance to change, and social problems resulting from change; mobile population; organizational and political problems among facilities, departments, and health agencies, etc.); and managerial problems (e.g. delays caused by large numbers of people involved in

decision making; choosing hardware prior to design of the
applications; no control over cost of operation, etc.).

Rural Problems

None of these problems is an absolute barrier to MIS diffusion,
merely an impediment. Likewise, none is limited to the rural setting,
although each is more serious in the rural situation. Technically,
low population densities mean that heavy (economical) loading of
a computer resource can only be achieved in the rural setting at
the expense of telecommunication costs over relatively long
distances. Reliability and back-up thus are compromised. Social
factors need not necessarily be more serious in rural areas, but
they usually are. Receptivity to advanced technological systems to
implement new service functions such as regional emergency medical
services has been an advantage; the relative lack of technologically
well trained local employees has been a counterbalancing
disadvantage.

Of the three documented barriers to MIS diffusion, the one most
serious lack in rural areas has been the frequent lack of
management capability. The development of all MIS's has required
sophisticated management to handle substantial fiscal resources
dedicated over a prolonged period of time. Successful MIS's have
had to solve complex management problems, both relating to the
internal affairs of the sponsoring organization and also the often
more complex issues of the relationships with external agencies of
the municipalities, states, federal regions, and private organizations. In the U.S., MIS's have tended to arise in major
metropolitan medical centers, frequently at the initiation of
university medical schools, and often with federal research
funding. Some countries have a well established and competent
health administration at the county or provincial level. This will
be a major advantage in implementing future information systems
for health care in rural areas.

Technical Obstacles and Future Rural MIS's

Two recent developments will tend to alleviate at least the
technical problems for rural MIS's. First, microprocessors appear
sufficient to perform a number of the MIS subsystem functions at
a local level, thus alleviating the previous economic demands for
heavy loading of large central computing facilities. Second,

electronic telecommunication networks, especially satellite-based communication systems, offer in the somewhat more distant future the possibility of eliminating ground distance as a bar to telecommunication efficiency.

Microprocessor technology offers remarkable reduction in the cost of computing capability (5). These devices are not yet able to substitute fully for a complete MIS. Consequently, one must think of them as performing individual MIS subsystem functions. Examples of potential microprocessor functions include the following: patient scheduling for a clinic or a medical service; hospital patient drug profiling; small drug information systems; EKG interpretation; clinical laboratory instrument control, test results reporting, and test interpretation; nurse scheduling; interrogative patient history; personal medical record; data encryption for privacy; data compression for storage efficiency.

It must be remembered that large central patient files cannot yet be maintained on microprocessors. Records for such files can be collected and edited by microprocessors but must ultimately be forwarded for storage on larger central machines. The extent to which the central machines can practically reconstruct appropriate subsets of the file for downstream processing and retrieval by the local microprocessors is not yet known, although the possibility is known. The general term which includes such concepts is "distributed processing" (3).

Communication networks now exist in the U.S. and elsewhere (2). These systems do much more than merely   send a computer signal over a distance. Recently competition between commercial networks has begun to focus on the extent to which value is added by the network to the message itself. This particular concept of value derives from the extent to which the network provides for enhanced reliability of the transmission (through such maneuvers as alternate routing and enhanced error detection and correction), for repackaging and compression of the message in order to effect savings through packet transmission, and the extent to which adaptation to different types of computer terminals and different computer data transmission protocols and speeds is provided automatically by the network rather than the originator of the message. In addition, most networks already ignore the number of miles over which a message is sent, basing their pricing simply on

either message size or connect time. The importance of such
practices for rural MIS's is obvious: they place the rural user on
a par with the metropolitan user in terms of the cost of accessing
special computer resources. Extension of commercial value-added
communication networks into the international and intercontinental
marketplace will take advantage of the space satellite
retransmission stations. Undoubtedly geo-political consideration
will dominate such arrangements between nations in the initial
phases, but in the end fundamental engineering considerations
assure that ground distance will become negligible as an economic
consideration, with potential benefit to rural health systems.

Both microprocessor developments and communication networks are
potentially advantageous to rural health systems, but their
effects are quite different. The microprocessors permit inexpensive
computation on a local basis. Their effect is centrifugal, tending
to permit information control at all levels of society. In contrast,
the modern communications systems increase the ease with which
information services and concommitant social control can be
effected from major central facilities. What balance will
ultimately be struck between these two trends is hard to predict.
From the point of view of those persons interested in improving
rural health care, it is highly desirable to initiate a new round
of formal medical experiments using both local microprocessors and
communication networks. In this way, there will be a medical basis
for influencing the outcome of the two new technologies.

References

1. Collen, M.F.: General Requirements. In Collen, M.F. (Ed.):
   Hospital Computer Systems, pp. 3-23. (New York: John Wiley and
   Sons 1974).

2. Cotton, I.W.: Computer Network Interconnection: Problems and
   Prospects. (Gaithersburg, MD.: National Bureau of Standards 1977).

3. Eckhouse, Jr., R.H., Stankovic, J.A., Van Dam, A.: Issues in
   distributed processing - An overview of two workshops.
   Computer 2 (1978) 22-26.

4. Lindberg, D.A.B.: The Growth of Medical Information Systems in
   the United States. (Lexington, Mass.: D.C. Heath and Company
   1979).

5. Noyce, R.N.: Microelectronics. Scient. Amer. 237, No. 3 (1977)
   62-69.

6. Rodnick, J.E., Wiederhold, G.: A review of automated ambulatory
   medical record systems in the U.S.: Charting services that
   are of benefit to the physician. In Shires, D.B. and Wolf H.
   (Ed.): MEDINFO 77, pp. 957-961. (Amsterdam: North-Holland 1977).

Health Information Systems for Large Communities

G. Griesser

Introduction

Structure, organization and function of a health information system (HIS) depend upon the health care system(s) to be serviced. Since a general model of a HIS in large communities does not exist, let me present the solution which has been chosen for Kiel. The presentation will be restricted to the information system of the Kiel University Hospital (KIEL KIS) (5, 7, 13) and that of the Association of Local Sick Funds of Schleswig-Holstein, named ADOSH (4). They are the main parts of the local interactive HIS (4, 8, 9, 19). However, it extends over a larger part of the country.

According to the distributed organization of health care in the Federal Republic of Germany, there is another health information system within the region, organized and managed by the Panel Doctors' Association of Schleswig-Holstein which has to perform the ambulatory health care. It operates as an off-line system communicating with KIEL KIS and ADOSH by exchange of data carriers.

Some health care data of the three systems are combined in the statistics of morbidity, issued by the State Bureau of Statistics of Schleswig-Holstein (4, 6). These statistics serve for hospital and ambulatory health care planning in connection with the population statistics (6, 14). In connection with hospital care planning in Schleswig-Holstein, it may be stated additionally that there is a rate of 5.4 beds per 1,000 inhabitants. This compares favourably with other parts of the Federal Republic of Germany.

If health information systems are discussed, then the more technical and organizational aspects may easily be overemphasized so that the human concern of the individual patient, being the central figure of any health care and information system, may be neglected. But we must not forget the human side in our considerations.

Description of Situation and Conditions

Geographic and Demographic Remarks.

Kiel is the capital of the most northern state of the Federal Republic of Germany, Schleswig-Holstein (Fig. 1), situated on the beautiful Kiel Fjord and especially known by the annual "Kiel Week" and the Olympic Sailing Games of 1972.

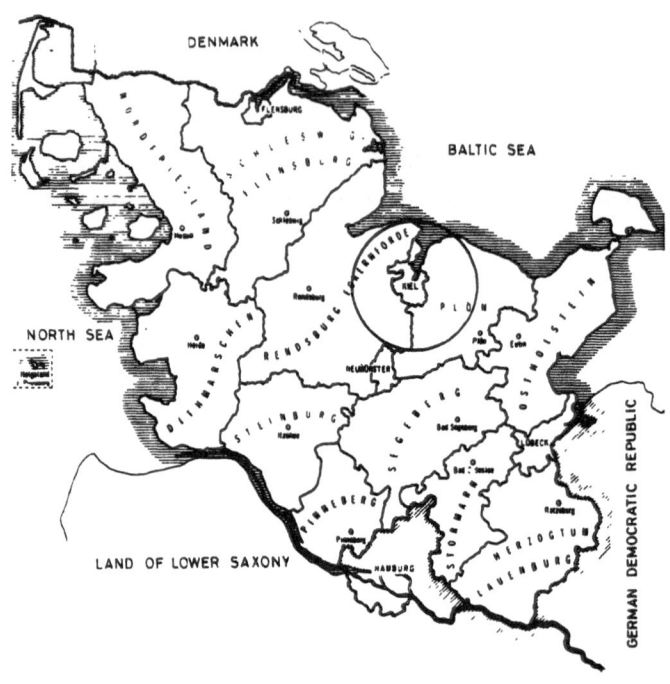

Fig. 1: Map of Schleswig-Holstein and Kiel
with its economic influence area

The town of Kiel.

The political community of Kiel has a population of about 271,000 inhabitants, while the economic zone includes about 360,000 persons. The main sectors of economy are shipbuilding, mechanical engineering and maritime trade, the latter due to the "Kiel Canal" connecting North and Baltic Sea. Kiel harbours a university now comprising some 12,800 students, with a Faculty of Medicine educating about 1,900 students of medicine and dental surgery.

Elements of hospital care.

There are the University Hospital containing 1,608 beds for acute
care, a middle-sized Community Hospital without surgical facilities
serving as teaching hospital, and some smaller private or
denominational hospitals. This contribution dealing with health
information systems is restricted to the University Hospital. Its
catchment population regarding all residencies of the country may be
seen from Table 1, comprising about 500,000 inhabitants of the

Table 1: Catchment population of Kiel hospital, related to all
residencies of Schleswig-Holstein (1)

RESIDENCE UNIT	POPULATION	CATCHMENT POPULATION FOR ALL DEPARTMENTS COMBINED
FLENSBURG	95 366	177 132
KIEL	271 042	502 368
LÜBECK	239 955	352 498
⋮	⋮	⋮
STEINBURG	132 543	119 799
STORMARN	159 142	107 194
	2 510 608	2 510 608

surroundings of Kiel (1). The number of discharges and bed-days of
this catchment population, broken down by age groups and sex, is

shown in <u>Fig. 2</u>. The calculation of the catchment population of a
hospital and its attraction rate may be seen from <u>Table 2</u>.

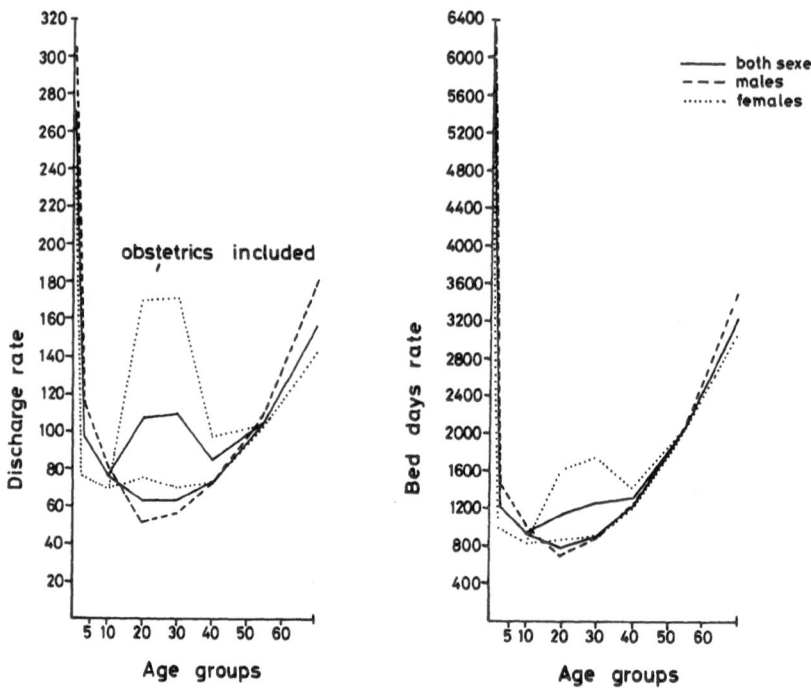

<u>Fig. 2</u>: Discharge rate and bed-days rate of the catch-
ment population of Kiel hospital (1)

In Table 2 column A indicates the number of annual admissions to the

Table 2: Catchment population and attraction rate of Kiel
         hospital, related to the population of the
         political community of Kiel

RESIDENCE UNIT	HOSPITAL KIEL(02) ALL DEPARTMENTS			RESIDENCE POPULATION	
	A	B	C	D	P
01	646	12,8%	12197	5051	95366
02	21353	97,9%	265436	21804	271042
03	121	6,0%	14452	2009	239955
15	674	15,4%	20457	4367	132543
16	49	2,9%	4609	1692	159142
TOTAL	37113	24,7%	621295	149971	2510608

hospital, column D the number of admissions out of column P = the
population of the residence unit (Kiel is presented in the second
row). Column B indicates the attraction rate in % of a hospital to
the population of a given residence unit. It is calculated B =
A x 100/D.

Column C shows the catchment population which is C = B x P.

The attraction rate of the Department of Surgery is depicted by
Fig. 3 (1, 14).

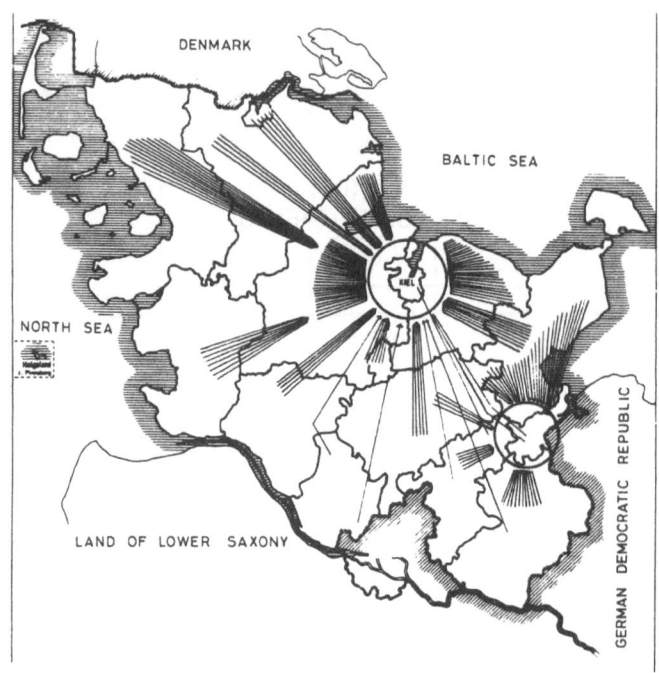

Fig. 3: Catchment area of the Department of
Surgery, Kiel University Hospital (1)

As shown by Table 3 derived from the KIEL KIS database, Kiel

Table 3: Residence units of the inpatients of Kiel University
Hospital, broken down by numbers of admission and
bed-days

FINZUGSGEBIETE DES GESAMTKLINIKUMS KIEL   1 9 7 7

PLANMAESSIGE BETTEN: TATSAECHLICH AUFGESTELLTE BETTEN:

	KREIS/LAND	PATIENTEN	PFLEGETAGE
1 =	FLENSBURG	856	12373
2 =	KIEL	16197	196436
3 =	LUEBECK	194	2119
4 =	NEUMUENSTER	1173	17145
51 =	DITHMARSCHEN	1114	15671
52 =	FLENSBURG-LAND	65	929
53 =	HZGT.LAUENBURG	100	1417
54 =	NORDFRIESLAND	1647	22666
55 =	OSTHOLSTEIN	1482	19765
56 =	PINNEBERG	116	1697
57 =	PLOEN	3891	47611
58 =	RENDSBURG/ECKERNFOERDE	5951	72005
59 =	SCHLESWIG	1685	21250
60 =	SEGEBERG	853	11105
61 =	STEINBURG	801	10865
62 =	STORMARN	68	686
	SCHLESWIG-HOLSTEIN ZUSAMMEN	36193	453740
90 =	HAMBURG	211	2237
95 =	ANDERE BUNDESLAENDER	1325	11850
97 =	DDR	6	110
98 =	AUSLAND	119	1188
	INSGESAMT	37554	469125

University Hospital serves the local population as well as that of
the region. The numbers of admissions and bed-days as well as the

average length of stay and the bed occupancy rate per annum from
1971 to 1977 are presented in Fig. 4.

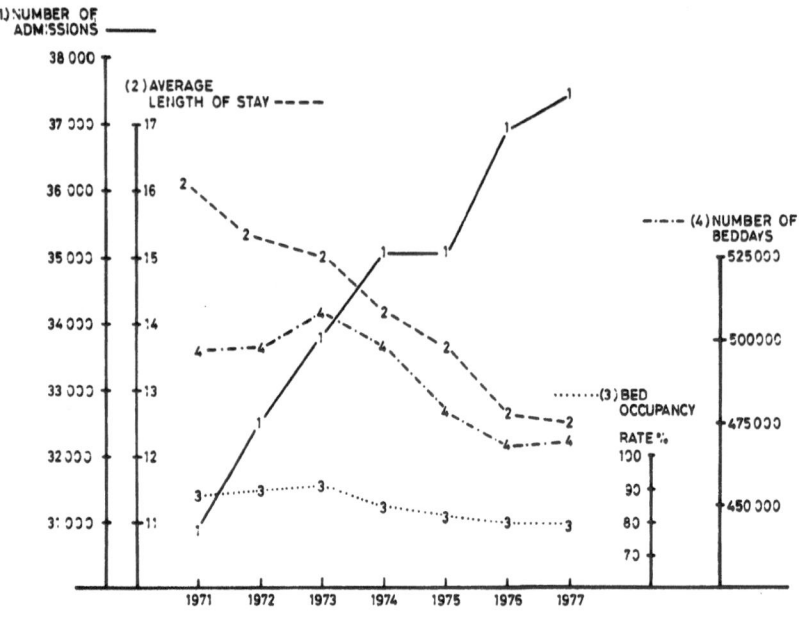

NUMBER OF ADMISSIONS (1),   AVERAGE LENGTH OF STAY (2),   BED OCCUPANCY RATE (3)
AND NUMBER OF BEDDAYS (4)   KIEL UNIVERSITY HOSPITAL 1971-1977

Fig. 4: Numbers of admissions and bed-days, average length
of stay and bed occupancy rate, Kiel University
Hospital, 1971-1977

As one can see, the numbers of admissions increased continuously,
whereas the numbers of bed-days decreased. This results in a
diminution of the average length of stay and of the bed occupancy
rate.

As shown in the following <u>Table 4</u> of the year 1977, the decrease of

Table 4: Departments, numbers of beds, admissions, bed-days
average lenght of stay and bed occupancy rate, Kiel
University Hospital 1977

Name of Department	Number of Beds	Number of Admissions/ Year	Number of Patient Days/ Year	Average Length of Stay in Days	Occupancy Rate%
Dept of Internal Medicine	220	6 637	76 304	11,6	95
Dept of Surgery	213	5 112	66 200	13,0	85
Women's Hospital (Obstetrics)	} 205	3 701	25 893	7,0	} 75
Women s Hospital (Gynaecology)		3 021	30 795	10,2	
Dept of Ophthalmology	103	3 243	31 786	10.0	84
Dept of Dermatology	120	1 910	36 418	20.0	83
Dept of Oto-Rhino-Laryngology	84	2 870	25 230	8.8	82
Children's Hospital	209	3 106	39 170	12.6	51
Dept of Psychiatry	185	2 174	58 839	27.1	87
Dept of Orthopaedics	90	1 906	30 063	15.8	91
Dept of Radiology	48	1 638	18 268	11.2	104
Dept of Dental Surgery	51	803	9 814	12.2	52
Dept of Neurosurgery	80	1 433	20 345	14.2	69
Total	1 608	37 554	469 125	12,5	79

Number of Admissions and Patientdays at the Kiel University Hospital 1977

the bed occupancy rate is caused mainly by a diminished utilization
of the Departments of Paediatrics, Dental Surgery and Neurosurgery.

The large Departments of Internal Medicine, Surgery and
Paediatrics are divided into three to four special divisions. Kiel
University Hospital employs 3,500 persons (physicians, nurses,
paramedical and administrative personnel, workers), i.e. 2.18
employees per bed.

The Health Information System of Kiel

General Remarks.

The expenditure caused by a computer-aided health information system is justified only if distinct aims have been defined as it was attempted in KIEL KIS and as it is shown by the following Table 5.

Aims of KIEL KIS

1. Improvement of Health Care by

    1. Better Health Care Information,
    2. Acceleration of Information Flow inside and outside the Hospital,
    3. Improvement of Steering and Control of the Hospital's Operation for

        1. Medical Care in Wards and Functional Units
        2. Management
        3. Medical Education
        4. Research,

    4. Better Planning.

2. Safeguard of Data Security
   (Privacy, Confidentiality, Data Integrity).

3. Rationalization of the Hospital's Operation by Automation of Routine Procedure of

    1. Management (Administrative, Medical),
    2. Requests of Medical Services outside the Wards,
    3. Control of (Medical) Services Rendered (Quality Control),
    4. Book-Keeping,
    5. Accounting,
    6. Statistical Service.

In this context it may be stated that the current costs of our system are very low. They amount to DM 1.05 per bed-day, including expenditure for the operators, the head of the computer center and the database administrator as well as the costs for electric current, air conditioning equipment, maintenance service by the computer manufacturers' technicians, paper, etc. The investment costs for the hardware equipment are not taken into account.

As presented elswewhere (8, 9, 19), the organizational advantages can only be fully gained in the medical services as well as in the management of large hospitals after the social environment of the hospital has been considered and integrated to the necessary extent, as it has been done by the interactive communication between KIEL KIS and ADOSH. On the other hand, Henney et al. (15) were able to demonstrate convincingly the improvement of communication within the care units themselves by a computer-supported hospital information system, an observation which meets our experience as well as that of others (3, 16, 17).

Kiel University Hospital Information System

KIEL KIS was designed as an integrated system with a centralized common database as mentioned by Schneider and Bengtsson (18). The underlying hardware equipment may be seen from Fig. 5

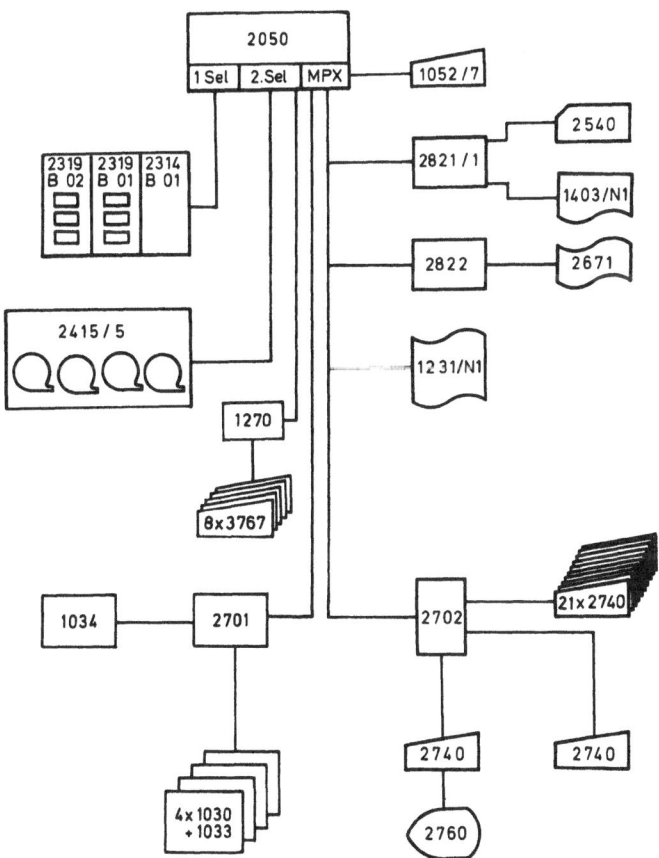

Fig. 5: Hardware equipment of KIEL KIS

At present there are 35 terminals for teleprocessing which provide multi-user/multi-purpose operation.

Additionally, there are several stand-alone dedicated systems in the Departments of Radiology (radiation planning, evaluation of nuclear-medical examinations) and of Paediatric Cardiology (ECG analysis, angio-cardio-densitometry), whereas the distributed laboratory information system is an integrated subsystem of KIEL KIS (2).

The structure of the database if presented by Fig. 6.

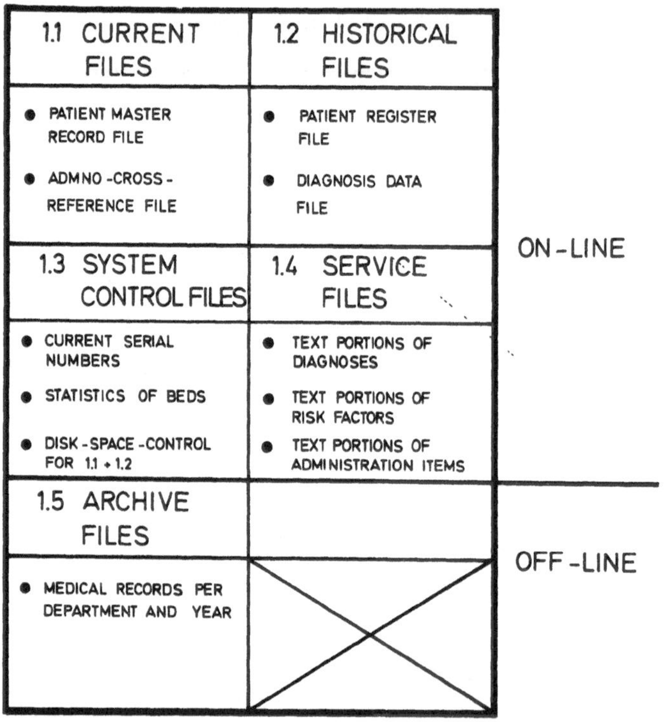

1.1 CURRENT FILES	1.2 HISTORICAL FILES	
• PATIENT MASTER RECORD FILE • ADM NO -CROSS - REFERENCE FILE	• PATIENT REGISTER FILE • DIAGNOSIS DATA FILE	
1.3 SYSTEM CONTROL FILES	1.4 SERVICE FILES	ON-LINE
• CURRENT SERIAL NUMBERS • STATISTICS OF BEDS • DISK-SPACE-CONTROL FOR 1.1 + 1.2	• TEXT PORTIONS OF DIAGNOSES • TEXT PORTIONS OF RISK FACTORS • TEXT PORTIONS OF ADMINISTRATION ITEMS	
1.5 ARCHIVE FILES		
• MEDICAL RECORDS PER DEPARTMENT AND YEAR		OFF-LINE

Fig. 6: Structure of the KIEL KIS database

The current files correspond to the temporary part of the database according to the IHF-study (18). The two historical files contain in the index part the patient register file and in the second part the diagnoses resulting from previous hospital stays.

The Structure of Health Care Data

Starting from a more comprehensive structure model of health care data (12), which is depicted in its various levels in Fig. 7,

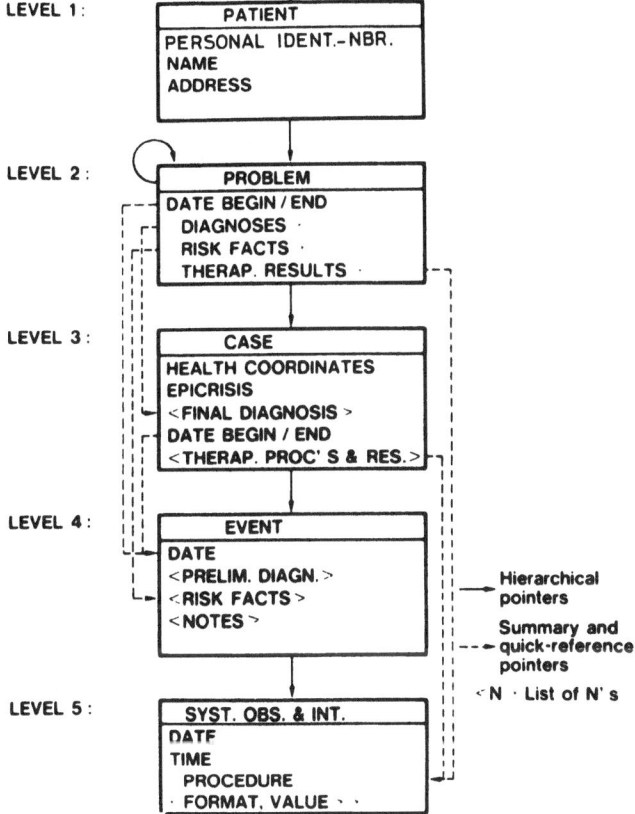

Fig. 7: Structure model of health care data

the various categories of data may be considered more generally in regard to the several classes of users as shown in Table 6.

Table 6: Institutions and classes of users according
to their information needs and categories of
health care data

INSTITUTION	USER	CATEGORIES OF DATA								
		P	S	M	D	R	A	RS	F	ST
HOSPITAL	PHYSICIAN	+	+	+	+	+	+	-	-	-
	NURSE	+	+	+	+	+	+	-	-	-
	MED. TECHNICIAN	+	-	(+)	(+)	-	-	-	-	-
	CLERK, ADMIN.	+	+	-	-	-	-	+	+	-
	HOSP. MANAGER	-	-	-	-	-	-	+	+	+
SICK FUND (HEALTH INSURANCE INSTITUTION)	CLERK	+	+	-	+	-	-	+	+	-
	MANAGER	-	+	-	-	-	-	-	+	+
	COMPANY DOCTOR	+	+	+	+	(+)	(+)	(+)	-	-
PANEL DOCTOR ASSOCIATION	PHYSICIAN	+	+	+	+	+	+	+	+	-
	NURSE-SECRETARY	+	+	-	+	-	-	+	+	-
	CLERK	-	+	-	-	-	-	+	+	-
	MANAGER	-	-	-	-	-	-	+	+	+
PUBLIC HEALTH SERVICE	PUBLIC HEALTH OFFICER	+	+	+	+	(+)	(+)	-	-	+
STATISTICAL OFFICE	CLERK	-	(+)	-	+	-	-	-	-	+
	MANAGER	-	(+)	-	+	-	-	-	-	+

The several users are classified according to their information needs,
depending on their functions and responsibilities, and set against
the categories of data.

The abbreviations mean:

- P = Personal data,
- S = Socio-medical data, such as family status, profession, employer, health insurance institution(s), family doctor, next of kin,
- M = Medical information (medical history, findings, laboratory test results, etc.),
- D = Diagnoses,
- R = Risk factors,
- T = Therapeutical measures,
- RS = Rendered Services, medical, to be placed to the sick funds' account,
- F = Financial data, i.e. money to be paid to the hospital,
- ST = STatistical data, rendered anonymous.

Table 7 gives a general survey of the flow of health care information

Table 7: Flow of health care information from the suppliers to the various users

FROM \ TO		PHYSICIAN (PANEL DOCTOR) 1	SPECIALIST (PANEL DOCTOR) 2	HOSPITAL 3	LOCAL SICK FUND 4	COMPANY DOCTOR 5	ASSOCIATION OF LOCAL SICK FUNDS 6	PANEL DOCTORS ASSOCIATION 7	STATE STATISTICAL OFFICE 8
PHYSICIAN (PANEL DOCTOR)	1		P.S, M. D,R,A	P. S,(M), D(R),A	P. S,D.	P. S,M, D,R,A	—	P. S,D. RS	—
SPECIALIST (PANEL DOCTOR)	2	P. S,M. R,D,A		P. S,M. D,R,A	P. S,D.	P. S,M. D,R,A	—	P. S,D. RS	—
HOSPITAL	3	P. S,M. D,A,R	P. S,M. D,RS,A		P. S,D. RS	—	—	—	(P),(S), D
LOCAL SICK FUND	4	P, S	P, S	P, S,F		P, S	ST	F	—
COMPANY DOCTOR	5	P. S,M. D	P. S,M. D	—	P. S,D		—	—	—
ASSOCIATION OF LOCAL SICK FUNDS	6	—	—	—	—	—		ST	ST
PANEL DOCTORS ASSOCIATION	7	F	F	—	P. S,D. RS	—	(P),(S), D ▲PREVENTION▼		—
STATE STATISTICAL OFFICE	8	—	—	(P),(S), D	—	—	—	—	

MATRIX OF INFORMATION FLOW IN A HEALTH CARE SYSTEM IN A LARGE COMMUNITY

according to suppliers and users, broken down by the various categories of data.

Tasks and Information Flow of KIEL KIS

Figure 8 shows the tasks performed by KIEL KIS for the medical

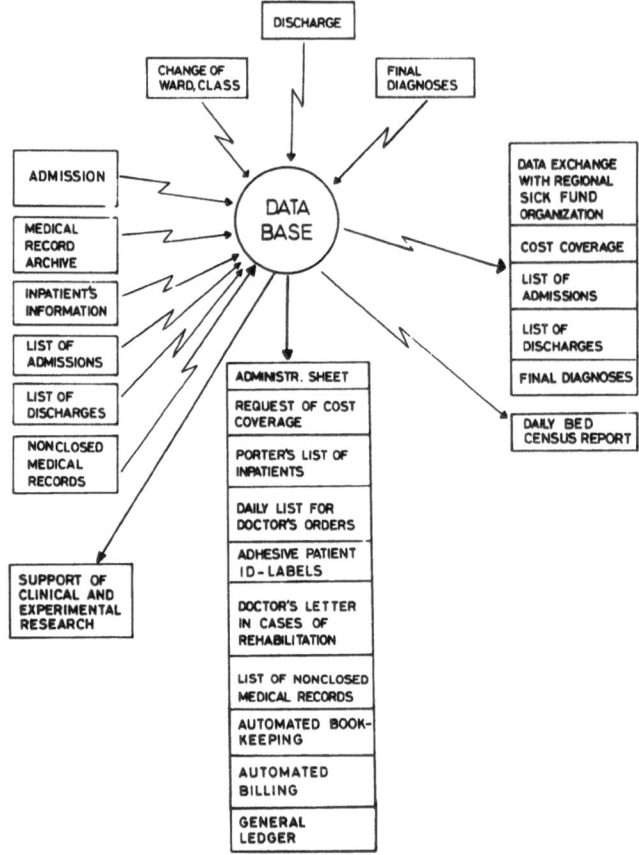

Fig. 8: Tasks of KIEL KIS

services as well as for managerial purposes including the interaction with ADOSH. The middle column below shows off-line applications, the other tasks being performed in one-line mode.

One can consider the information flow within a hospital as a circulation of data, particularly if one takes into account that at least 25 percent of all inpatients are re-admitted within one to three years.

This circulation of hospital care information is depicted in **Fig. 9**.

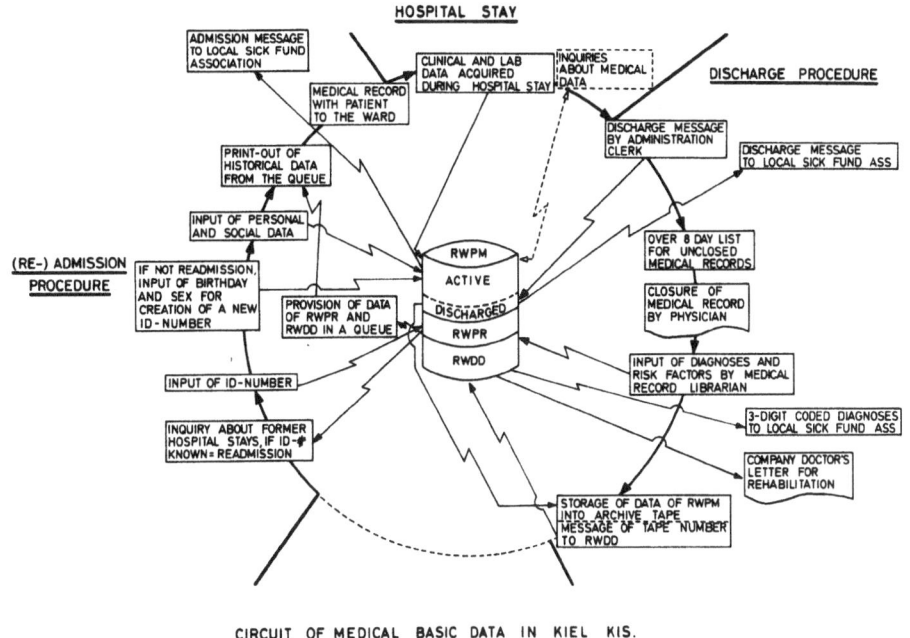

CIRCUIT OF MEDICAL BASIC DATA IN KIEL KIS.

Fig. 9: Circulation of health care information inside and
outside KIEL KIS

The connection of KIEL KIS with ADOSH

As mentioned elsewhere (5, 8, 19), a more or less complete benefit
from rationalization by computer-aided health information systems
could not be achieved before the on-line connection of KIEL KIS with
ADOSH, the sick fund information system of Schleswig-Holstein, had
been established. This interactive communication results in a nearly
"paperless administration" providing either partner with more
complete information within a minimum of time which is for the benefit
of inpatients and the hospital management as well as of the sick-funds.
The sick fund company doctors are included in the exchange of health
care information. The benefits gained by the connection of the two
systems may be illustrated by the fact that about 55 percent of the
inpatients, treated in the Kiel University Hospital, are members of
one of the local sick funds of our country. This means that the

principle of paperless administration is applied to more than fifty
percent of the inpatients. Their data are handled by the ADOSH
teleprocessing network system.

If one regards invoices and payment, i.e. money, as a kind of
information as shown in Tables 6 and 7, further profit is gained by
either organizational partner by the automated accounting procedure
on the part of the hospital and the automated payment on the part of
the sick funds, performed by off-line exchange of storing media.

Identification and Information Linkage

There is some difficulty in the identification of the elements of a
comprehensive health care and information system unless a population
number, as in some countries, has been introduced. Since such an
introduction failed in the Federal Republic of Germany for various,
mainly political reasons, we had to use alternative methods which
allow the unique identification of the inpatients in KIEL KIS and
of the insured persons in ADOSH.

The principle of person- and case-related identification, which links the numerous data of the inpatients, and the insurance-related identification is shown by <u>Table 8</u>.

<u>Table 8</u>: Identification of inpatients (person, case) and of the members of local sick funds

PATIENT IDENTIFICATION

PERSON-RELATED (PK) = | D,D,M,M,Y,Y| S | N,N,N,N|F|

DATE OF BIRTH   SEX SERIAL   DUMMY
                       NUMBER   CHAR.

CASE-RELATED   = | D,D|Y,Y|N,N,N,N|
(ADMISSION NUMBER)

DEPT YEAR   SERIAL
NUMBER   NUMBER

SICK FUND-RELATED = | D,D,M,M,Y,Y|N,N,N| N | S|C|
(SOCIAL INSURANCE NUMBER)

DATE OF BIRTH   SURNAME FIRST SEX CHECK
                             NAME,   DIGIT

INITIALS CODED

The unique person-related identifier (PK) and the case-related identification, i.e. the admission number are generated automatically by KIEL KIS. PK is generated once only at the first admission and used as a link to the case(s) of re-admission(s).

Since the structures of the person- and the insurance-related identifiers are similar, the unique identification of a person is ensured in either direction from and to the hospital if the inpatient's name is used additionally.

Problems of Integrated and Connected Health Information Systems

Coordination and Cooperation.

A 1,600-bed hospital is in reality a large-scale enterprise and eventually a rather sensitive organism. Therefore, the disturbance of the daily work of hospital care must be avoided by introducing a computer-aided information system with its inherent alterations of some organizational procedures handed down for decades. Therefore, KIEL KIS has been introduced step by step taking into consideration the special conditions which varied from department to department. However, the leading principle of standardization of the administrative and managerial tasks to be performed at the wards as well in the admission offices had to be observed. This was not true for medical records sheets and other forms only, but for the dictionaries used for the classification of diagnoses, laboratorial services and therapeutical measures.

For these reasons, some preparatory work had to be done by our department in order to create the organizational preconditions. This was possible due to a close cooperation with the clinical departments. But,on the other hand,the medical staff, first of all the head physicians of the departments and divisions, and the hospital nurses had to be convinced and motivated to adopt a new and unknown system. One argument of objection was the fear of being controlled by the computer in all steps to be taken. This objection cannot be completely disregarded because it is true to some extent, as one target of an integrated and comprehensive information system is to give the underlying health care system and its medical and administrative management more transparency with regard to all services rendered.

Since physicians are inclined to be rather individualistic which may lead to pure stubbornness, it was a difficult task to be solved. In this connection, the famous "human factor" must be kept in mind because a man-computer-system, like a computer-aided HIS, cannot operate smoothly and effectively without an adapted human behaviour. Therefore, some careful and cautious education was needed in order to overcome a certain preliminary opposition. But once the participants (physicians, nurses, administrative personnel) in a HIS can see the benefits brought by the system, they are willing to neglect and forget the putative disadvantages. For these reasons, KIEL KIS was designed from the very beginning to regard the concerns of all groups of personnel involved in KIEL KIS and the connected

ADOSH system.

The Issue of Privacy and Confidentiality

Computer-aided HIS are supposed to threaten the intimacy of the patient-physician relationship. But, in my opinion, it is a very shallow consideration of the problem, the importance of which cannot be denied. For reasons of time it cannot be discussed in detail, but there is a wealth of literature on the subject.

Doubtless, data protection measures are necessary in order to safeguard data security. That means that data integrity must be guaranteed as well as the protection of confidential health care data against any unintentional or deliberate misuse.

However, when you go deeper into the problem, you will find that the menace to privacy is not originally caused by the application of the computer in health care. On the contrary, the environmental conditions of the conventional health care systems have been altered in course of time, due to the introduction of systems of social security and by uncontrolled channels leading outside the proper health care sphere into information areas little or not related to health care as shown, for instance, by Westin (21).

System analyses of conventional health care systems, performed carefully and unbiasedly, will show numerous loopholes threatening privacy and confidentiality. They must be recognized and plugged before computer-supported HIS can be implemented.

In this connection, it may be emphasized that a broad spectrum of data protection measures is offered in a carefully designed HIS by hardware precautions, software techniques and organizational rules (10, 11, 21).

An important precondition of effective data protection is, inter
alia, the classification of data according to their sensitivity and
of users according to their information needs according to their
functions and responsibilities. Table 9 shows such a categorization
of data in a simplified manner.

Table 9: Categories of health care data
and sensitivity classes

CATEGORY OF DATA	ABBRE- VIATION	SENSITIVE CATEGORY			
		N	S	VS	HS
PERSONAL	P	+			
SOCIO-MEDICAL	S	+			
MEDICAL	M			+	+
DIAGNOSIS	D			+	+
RISK FACTORS	R		+		
ACTIVITIES	A			+	
RENDERED MEDICAL SERVICES	RS		+		
FINANCIAL	F		+		
STATISTICAL (ANONYMOUS)	ST	+	+		

Categories of Health Care Data and Categories of Sensitivity

N = NORMAL . DATA ACCESSIBLE TO ALL PARTICIPANTS IN A HIS, SUBJECTED TO THE OBLIGATION OF CONFIDENTIALITY

S = SENSITIVE. DATA ACCESSIBLE TO DEFINED GROUPS OF USERS ONLY

VS=VERY SENSITIVE: DATA ACCESSIBLE TO SELECTED EXPLICITLY AUTHORIZED GROUPS OF USERS

HS=HIGHLY SENSITIVE. DATA ACCESSIBLE ONLY BY PATIENTS CONSENT

However, the human factor mentioned before must not be neglected
in the issue of data security. The technical and organizational
protection measures can only operate effectively if all participants
in a computer-aided HIS are educated in such a way that they are
always aware of their duty of confidentiality. Therefore, the
ethical conduct (20) of the personnel involved in immediate and
mediate health care is an unalterable prerequiste of data security.

A further precondition is the informed consent (21) of the patient
whose health care information is being handled. The duty of
confidentiality, i.e. to keep secret the patient's health care data,
and the extent of the informed consent depend upon the laws or

other legal regulations of data security which apply to the
location of a given HIS.

Benefits and Drawbacks of a Computer-Supported Health Information System

In summing up, benefits and disadvantages of a health information
system are presented in the following scheme.

	Benefits	Drawbacks
Patient	1. Improvement of Health Care 2. Decreased Length of Stay 3. Improvement of Medical Decision Making	1. Menace to Privacy
Hospital	1. Improvement of Organizational Control and Survey 2. Improvement of Information Flow 3. Transparency of the Hospital Flow 4. Rationalization of Internal Organization 5. Quality Control of Health Care Data 6. Automated Book-keeping 7. Acceleration of Accounting	1. Cost of EDP, Investment in Hardware, Current EDP Operation 2. Certain Rigidity of Hospital. Operation by Strict Rules of the "Computer Game" 3. Menace to Hospital Privacy 4. Supervision of Hospital Staff
Sick Fund	1. Improvement of Health Care 2. Acceleration of Information Flow 3. Decrease of Costs of Hospital Care 4. Rationalization of Processing of Health Care Data	1. Loss of Interest
Government	1. Improvement of Information for Hospital Planning 2. Improvement of Survey of Health Status of Population	

As one can see, the benefits offered by a computer-supported HIS
to the various persons or institutions outweigh the disadvantages.
Some of those, such as the menace to privacy and an incongruous
rigidity of the system which will lead to a continuous harassment
of the users, can be avoided if the system is planned, designed
and organized carefully and considerately in regard to the tasks to
be performed and to the justified demands of the users working in
health care.

References

1. Bridgeman, R.F.: Hospital Utilization. An International Study.
   Unpublished, 1975.

2. Carstensen, K., Fischer, T., Griesser, G., Dörner, K.:
   Development and Test of a Laboratory System as Part of an
   Integrated Hospital Information System. Proceed. Ann. Conference
   Med. Inform., Toulouse, March 13-17, 1978.

3. Collen, M.F. (Edit.): Hospital Computer Systems. Wiley & Sons,
   New York 1974.

4. Griesser, G.: Wie können unsere Daten sozialmedizinisch ausge-
   wertet werden? Ortskrankenkasse 54 (1972) 783-793.

5. Griesser, G.: Das Klinik-Informationssystem des Klinikums der
   Christian-Albrechts-Universität zu Kiel (KIEL KIS). Universität
   Kiel 1975.

6. Griesser, G.: General Statistics and Hospital Information. In
   Kool, G.A. (Edit.): Hospital Statistics and a Minimum Basic
   Data Set, pp. 63-81. Netherlands Institute for Preventive
   Medicine, Leyden 1976.

7. Griesser, G.: Presentation und Use of Medical Basic Information
   in KIEL KIS. In Egmond, J. van, Vries-Robbé, P.F. de, Levy,
   A.H. (Eds.): Information Systems for Patient Care, pp. 205 - 220.
   North-Holland, Amsterdam 1976.

8. Griesser, G.: A Hospital Information System in the Environment of
   the Regional Insurance System - not just a Hypothetical Model.
   In Masè, E., Collen, M.F., Gorini, S. (Eds.): The Computer in
   Health Care Systems in Some European Countries and in the United

States, pp. 85-98. Piccin Medical Books, Padua 1976.

9. Griesser, G.: Kommunikation zwischen einem Krankenhaus- und einem Versicherungs-Informationssystem. In Wagner, G., Köhler, C.O. (Hrsg.): Interaktive Datenverarbeitung in der Medizin, S. 113-121. Schattauer, Stuttgart 1976.

10. Griesser, G.: (Edit.): Realization of Data Protection in Health Information Systems. North-Holland, Amsterdam 1977.

11. Griesser, G.: Technical Aspects of Data Protection in Health Information Systems. In Shires, D.B., Wolf, H. (Eds.): MEDINFO 77, pp. 723-728. North-Holland, Amsterdam 1977.

12. Griesser, G., Jainz, M., Sauter, K., Schneider, W.: A Data Structure Model for a Health Information System. Comput. Progr. Biomed. 6 (1976) 171-177.

13. Griesser, G., Jainz, M., Straach, H.-P., Carstensen, K., Voss, J.D.: Kiel University Hospital Information System. In Shires, D.B., Wolf, H. (Eds.): MEDINFO 77, p. 1047. North-Holland, Amsterdam 1977.

14. Griesser, G., Hedderich, J.: Some Considerations on Multivariate Hospital Statistics. Proceed. Ann. Conference on Medical Informatics, Toulouse, Mach 13-18, 1978.

15. Henney, C.R., Bosworth, R., Brown, N., Crooks, J.: Can a Computer Improve Communication in the Ward Area? In Shires, D.B., Wolf, H. (Eds.): MEDINFO 77, pp. 935-956, North-Holland, Amsterdam, 1977.

16. Peterson, H.: The Stockholm County Medical Information System. Proceed. Symposium on Computer Information System in Health Care, Moscow 1975, pp. 27-39. Sperry Univac, London 1976.

17. Reichertz, P.L.: The Medical System Hannover (MSSH). In Collen, M.F. (Edit.): Hospital Computer Systems, pp. 598-661. Wiley & Sons, New York 1974.

18. Schneider, W., Bengtsson, S., Anderson, J., Kästner, V., Lamson, B., Pratt, A., Reichertz, P., Robinson, A., Sandblad, B., Spencer, W.: The Application of Computer Techniques in Health Care with Special Regard to Hospitals. Comput. Progr. Biomed. 5 (1976) 169-250.

19. Straach, H.-P., Griesser, G.: Interaction of a Hospital Infor-
    mation System with a Regional Sick Fund Information System.
    In Anderson, J., Forsythe, J.M. (Eds.): MEDINFO 74, pp. 533-537.
    North-Holland, Amsterdam 1974.

20. Vallbona, C., Beggs-Baker, S.: Data Protection in a Community
    Medicine Environment. In Griesser, G. (Edit.): Realization of
    Data Protection in Health Information Systems, pp. 45-54.
    North-Holland, Amsterdam 1977.

21. Westin, A.L.: Computers, Health Records and Citizen Rights.
    U.S. Nat. Bur. Stand. Monogr. 157 (1976).

Health Problems of Low Income Communities

C. Vallbona

Introduction

In the majority of large cities of the Western World, there is a
significant proportion of low income persons whose health problems
are dealt with through publicly funded health care systems. The
relative size of the low income population varies from country to
country and from city to city within each country. The 1970
census of the USA showed a national average of 10.7% poor families,
the percentage being higher in the rural areas (15%) than in the
cities (9%).

The percentages fluctuate according to the economic conditions of
the country which in turn dictate the migration of significant
numbers of low income families from one area (urban or rural)
to the other.

If we take into account that many cities have a total population
in excess of one million, it is evident that the health care for
the poor of these cities becomes a major concern and deserves
special analysis.

In this report, we will:

a) review the health problems that are highly prevalent among
the disadvantaged urban poor and which require specific
community health interventions;

b) analyze the factors which place the poor at greater health
risks than the general population;

c) point out the characteristics of the publicly funded health
care systems which lead to serious deficits;

d) analyze some technological applications which are being
evaluated for their potential effectiveness in the
prevention and control of specific community health
problems.

In our presentation, we will follow the analytic approaches of
community medicine, a discipline that assesses the health status
of community groups, analyzes the community health problems and
seeks solutions through organization of health care delivery
systems that are responsive to the needs of individual patients
and of the community as a whole. In general, these community health
problems can be dealt with adequately at the primary care level.
Primary care includes the services rendered to individuals who
present health problems that are rather common and do not require
complex facilities beyond those available in ambulatory care
settings. The primary care provider is a family practitioner, a
general pediatrician, or a general internist. Typical primary care
settings are physicians' offices, group practices, hospital
outpatient departments, emergency rooms, and community health
centers. It is at the primary care level where new technological
applications hold greatest promise of making a significant impact
on the state of health of a community.

Prevalent Health Problems among the Urban Poor

It is well known that age-specific mortality due to certain
conditions is greater among the disadvantaged poor than in the
general population. Similarly, the level of disability brought
about by certain chronic illnesses is significantly greater in the
low income than in the high income groups. Such a relationship
as it has been established for six activity-limiting conditions
is shown in Figure 1.

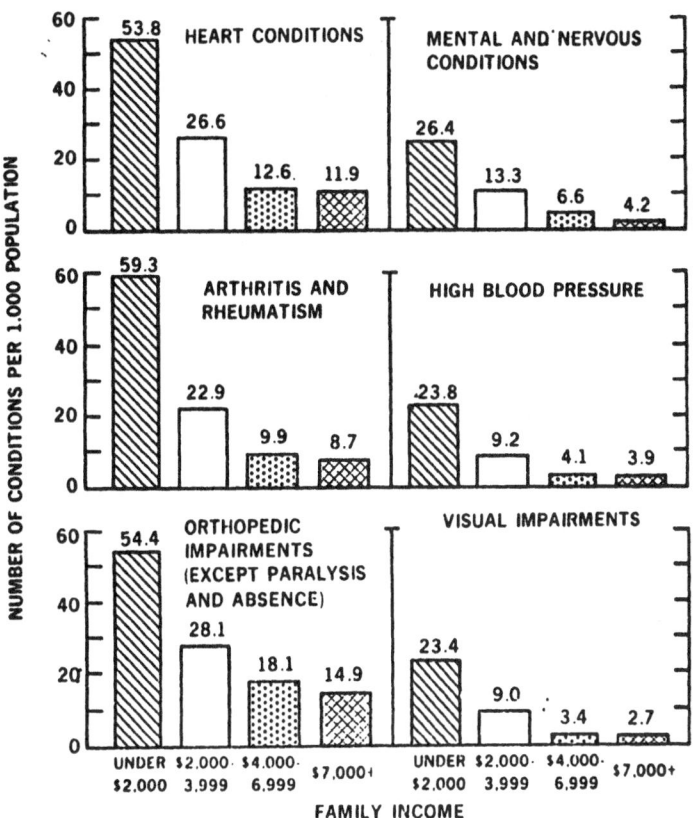

Fig.1: Activity-limiting conditions, by income 1964

The problems that we have encountered most commonly among children
of low income families include prematurity and infant respiratory
distress, probably because low income pregnant mothers are at
greater risk of having premature infants who in turn are more prone
to develop infant respiratory distress. Another common problem is
the low immunization level of children, especially those of
preschool age. Gastrointestinal infections, parasitosis, and
impetigo also constitute common problems which occur in greater
prevalence among the children of disadvantaged families. Child abuse
has emerged in the last few years as a significant community health
problem in several countries and is occurring with greater
frequency among low income families.

Health problems that are more prevalent amont the low income adults
are, e.g., complications of pregnancy that account for a high
percentage of visits to a primary care facility. The problems of
greatest concern to us are those of chronic illnesses such as
hypertension, ischemic heart disease, diabetes, and obesity which
constitutes the greatest challenges to community health
professionals. Venereal diseases and drug addiction complete the
picture of the problems that deserve special attention although
they are certainly not unique to low income populations.

Risk Factors

It is important that we analyze those factors that make the low
income persons more susceptible to the above mentioned health
problems than the general population. These factors should be
analyzed within the context of an individual's socio-economic
condition, his health attitudes, and his ethnicity.

1. Socio-economic Conditions. The following list includes the risk
   factors that are related to the socio-economic conditions under
   which most of the low income persons live:

   - Crowding

   - Inadequate sanitation

   - Inappropriate nutrition habits

   - Physical stress during work

   - Mental stresses

2. Health Attitudes. Factors associated with the attitudes that low
   income persons have toward health include:

   - Fatalistic attitude toward illness: chance, trial
     or punishment
   - Inadequate awareness of early signs of illness
   - Inadequate awareness of risk habits: smoking
   - Crisis care rather than prevention
   - Poor compliance with prescribed treatments
   - Adherence to folk medicine

Some of these attitudes make them more vulnerable to certain
health problems because the patients do not seek competent
health care when they should and, as a result, it is extremely
difficult to achieve the desired levels of disease control at
the community level.

3. Ethnicity. In multiracial communities, poverty occurs more often
   in certain ethnic groups who are particularly susceptible to
   specific health problems because of a genetic predisposition
   (e.g., sickle cell disease among blacks). Similarly, certain
   health attitudes which run counter to good health practices
   are ingrained in certain population groups (such as the belief
   in folk medicine which we find among uneducated Mexican
   Americans).

   It is important that we understand clearly how an individual's
   attitudes or beliefs are major determinants of his/her health
   seeking behavior. The health belief model proposed by Becker
   et al. ( ) shown in Figure 2 illustrates the relationships
   between demographic and socio-psychological variables, perceived
   health threats, cues for action, and the likelihood that a
   patient take preventive health action.

Deficiencies in the Health Care System

Donabedian ( ) has identified three basic components in a health
care system: structure, process, and outcome. These three
components provide a suitable framework to assess the extent to
which any health care system is responsive to the needs of the
community (or population at risk) which it is purported to serve.
Figure 3 depicts this model.

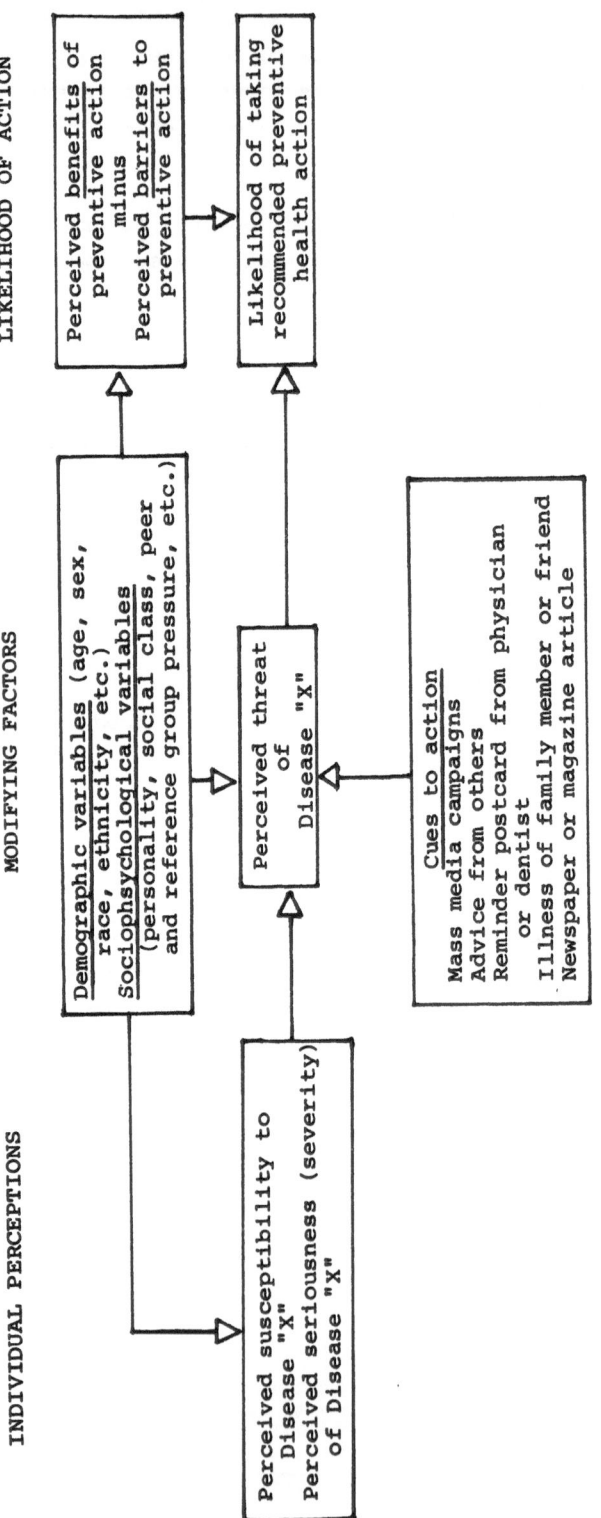

Fig. 2: Original "Health Belief Model" as predictor of preventive health behavior

HEALTH CARE SYSTEM

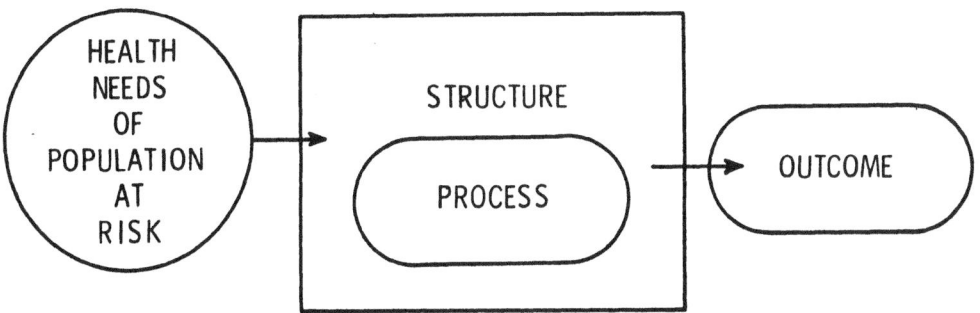

Fig. 3:Basic components of a health care system

The structure refers to the setting in which health services are rendered and the organization which is responsible for such services. The population served by the system, the physical facilities, the medical staff, administrative personnel, the political structure responsible for the establishment of health policies and the organization which finances the care process are the essential elements of the structure.

The process is the set of activities that take place when services are provided. Within the process, we must consider the flow of individuals through the system, the volume and types of services rendered, the flow of information generated in the care process, health manpower inputs, economic inputs, etc.

The outcome relates to the impact that the structure and the process have on the state of health of the individuals or community groups who utilize the health care system. We usually express outcomes in terms of mortality or morbidity but we should consider also other outcomes such as the functional status of the individuals who have been treated by the health system.

Deficiencies in the structure. The following list shows several aspects of the structure of publicly funded health care systems which jeopardize, rather than facilitate, the control of many community health problems that we encounter in low income populations.

- Health policy affected by politics
- Complex bureaucracy
- Inadequate incentives for health professionals
- Restricted funding
- Highly mobile patient population

We have singled out the fact that health policies are affected by politics, that there is complex bureaucracy, that health professionals have inadequate incentives to provide quality care and that in many circumstances the funds allocated to community health programs are somewhat restricted.

Deficiencies in the process. The peculiar characteristics of the health care process which account for most of its serious deficiencies include:

- Demand in excess of capacity
- Contact with numerous health professionals
- Inadequate physician/patient relationship
- Redundancy of services
- Insufficient coordination of activities
- General inefficiency

In general, the demand exceeds the capacity of the system, the patient must establish contact with numerous health professionals, and this leads to inadequate physician/patient relationships. As a result, there is redundancy of services, insufficient coordination of activities, and a general gross inefficiency.

Deficiencies in the outcome. Most public health care systems do not have clearly pre-established objectives. Even when they are clearly formulated, they often remain unfulfilled and,since the cost of services may be high because of gross inefficiencies, the overall performance of the system is poor.

Applications of Technology in Primary Care

Sophisticated new technologies have been utilized extensively in medicine for the last 30 years. Although their greatest impacts, both positive and negative, have been felt at the secondary or tertiary care hospitals, recent technological developments have been introduced at the primary care level and they hold great promise of facilitating the control of specific health problems in low income communities.

1. Goals. The following list, by no means exhaustive, shows the major goals of applications of technology at the primary care level:

    - Promote general health education

    - Increase awareness of risk factors

    - Improve availability of and accessibility
      to preventive services

    - Facilitate delivery of emergency care

    - Enhance efficiency of health care information systems

    - Contain the cost of care within pre-established limits

    - Monitor adequately the outcome of health services.

We believe that these goals are realizable and, although much developmental work is required before widespread implementation of some new technological developments, we are convinced that the benefits derived in community health will be remarkable.

Through technology we should be able to promote general health education and increase the level of awareness of low income persons about the major risk factors in order to achieve positive action toward prevention of illness. Widespread availability of preventive services and easy accessibility to them requires mobilization of the technological resources required to facilitate early detection of illness or to assess with precision the type and degree of functional disability. Prompt delivery of emergency care is a major need in low income urban areas. Consequently, it is necessary to make full use of technology to achieve deployment of effective emergency medical systems wherever and whenever they are needed. Health care information systems in ambulatory settings are also absolutely necessary to

improve the efficiency of the care process, and to contain the
cost of ambulatory care within the limits of available
resources. Finally, it is important that we make available to
physicians and health care administrators the technology that
is required to monitor adequately the outcome of health
services provided at the primary care level.

2. Examples. We have acquired experience in the application of
health care technology in the prevention and control of
cardiovascular diseases in low income neighborhoods of Houston,
Texas. Most of this experience has been obtained through the
National Heart and Blood Vessel Research and Demonstration
Center of Baylor College of Medicine which is supported by a
grant from the National Heart, Lung and Blood Institute.

The metropolitan Houston area has a population slightly above two
million. Approximately 250,000 individuals are considered to be
medically indigent and most of them live in rather circumscribed
areas scattered throughout the city. Figure 4 shows the geographic

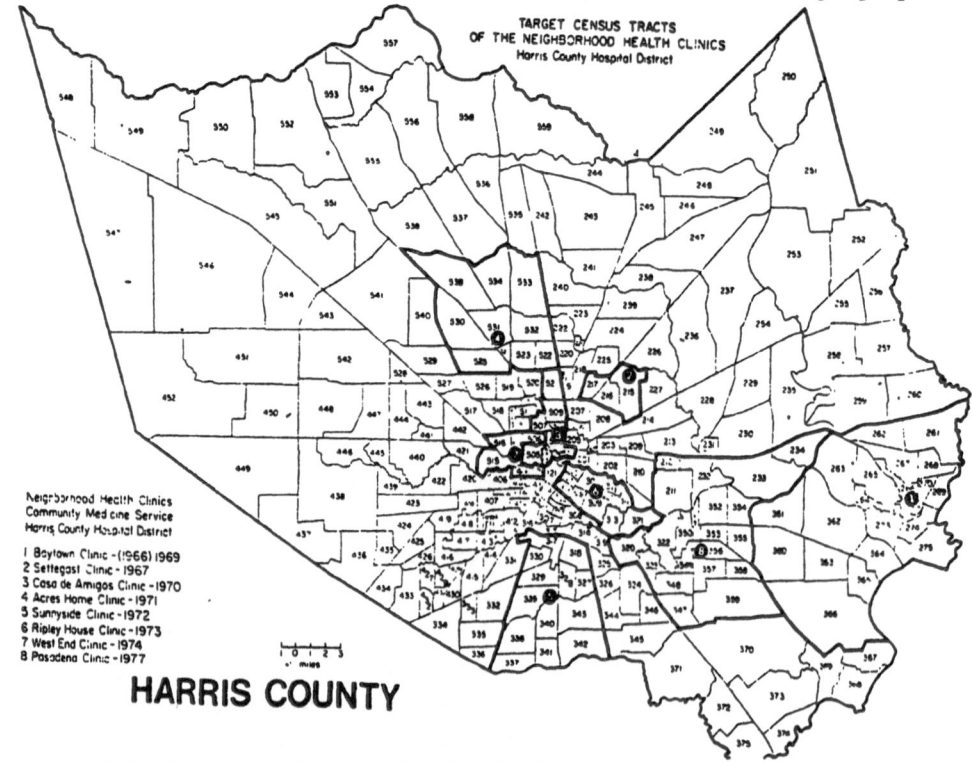

Fig. 4: Harris County Hospital District

distribution of the low income groups and the location of eight
community health centers which the Harris County Hospital District
has established in collaboration with Baylor's Department of
Community Medicine. The profile of health problems encountered in
these scattered communities is in agreement with the data
presented above.

The Division of Control and Demonstration and the Division of
Education of Baylor's Heart Center have established community
health awareness programs using public media to promote good health
habits of the low income population, especially those that have the
greatest risk of developing cardiovascular problems.

In order to train adequately as many community persons as possible
in the handling of emergency situations that result from cardiac
or respiratory arrest, we have established training programs on the
techniques of cardiopulmonary resuscitation. We make use of
specially instrumented mannequins that allow the instructor to
monitor the effectiveness of the trainee's efforts to achieve
ventilation and appropriate cardiac output.

Collen and coworkers ( ) have demonstrated the cost-effectiveness
of submitting patients to an annual automated multiphasic screening.
We have screened systematically all our patients for those illnesses
that are prevalent in the populations served by our community
health centers.

The numerous medical emergencies that occur in the city of Houston
are handled through a municipal emergency medical system which
makes use of telemetry-equipped ambulances and helicopters.
Specially trained emergency medical technicians can thus arrive at
the scene of an emergency within a few minutes of a call to a
central dispatcher. The technicians can institute life-saving
procedures while cardiac function is telemetered to a central base
station located in the Emergency Center of Ben Taub General Hospital
in the Texas Medical Center. The patient will be transferred
to the nearest community hospital which can handle the specific
problem that the patient presents.

For the last five years, we have worked extensively on the development of a computerized ambulatory care information system which
has been implemented in our community health centers. We believe
that the system, described later on, has been of major usefulness to

our primary care physicians and to the administrative personnel of
the community health centers.

A list of the specific examples of technological applications which
we have used in our community includes:

- Media campaigns to promote good health habits
- Media campaigns targeted to specific risks
- Simulation of life-saving treatment
- Automated health screening systems
- Telemetry-equipped ambulances and helicopters
- Ambulatory care information systems

Ambulatory Care Information Systems

The major objectives of computerized ambulatory care information
systems are:

- Facilitate flow and use of personal health-illness
  information
- Expedite the care process to meet increasing demands
- Study changes in the prevalence of community health
  problems
- Monitor the volume and cost of services rendered
- Analyze productivity of health professionals
- Assess the quality of care
- Evaluate the impact of specific health care strategies
- Provide a data base for health services research
- Assist in the education of primary care professionals

Our experience indicates that these objectives can be realized
through the application of simple techniques of medical informatics.

Indeed, a computerized ambulatory care information system can be of
great assistance in facilitating the flow and use of the health-
illness information contained in a summary of a patient's ambulatory
medical record. If this summary is made readily available to the
authorized community health center personnel, the care process can
be expedited and the demands for service can be met with greater

ease. By interrogating the data base of individual records, one can study changes in the prevalence of community health problems and assess the extent to which normal seasonal variations   occur. It is important also to assess on a quantitative basis the volume and cost of services rendered in order to set up objectives for containing or optimizing such costs. Since the data base contains information of professional services rendered, it is possible also to analyze the productivity of health professionals and the quality of care rendered to the patients. The evaluation of the impact of specific health care strategy is facilitated through an appropriate ambulatory care information system. Lastly, if the system includes a carefully edited data base, it is possible to conduct a variety of health services research activities and to facilitate the education of medical students and allied health professionals.

In 1973, we began the development of a computerized information system for one of our community health centers (Casa de Amigos). As a result of our development, we have produced a practical and relatively inexpensive method of storing in a computer a summary of the ambulatory record of all persons who are seen in the center. The summary document is referred to as the Health-Illness Profile and contains the following information:

      a) a list of all the patients active problems;
      b) a list of current medications;
      c) the services rendered at the last visit;
      d) the most important health risks; and,
      e) demographic and identification data.

A health-illness profile is generated automatically by the computer after each patient visit.

The computerized data base of updated profiles of all patients seen in the community health center has given opportunity to the physician in chief and to the clinic manager to assess periodically the effectiveness and efficiency of the care process. As a result of the successful implementation of this information system for one community health center, we have designed a similar system for the whole network of eight community health centers. The new system will provide for merging of the medical data base with the data base collected on each patient for fiscal purposes. As a result, we will be in a better position to make in-depth economic analyses of the care process and relate it to its outcomes.

At each community health center, we have an intelligent terminal operated by a clerk who extracts from the medical record the most relevant medical and administrative data. Specially designed source documents facilitate the extraction. The data are entered into diskettes and at the end of the day a summary report is printed which summarizes the services rendered to all the patients at the center on that day. All the diskettes are transferred to a central computer facility for storage and generation of a data base which has been specially designed to store the health-illness profiles of the more than 100,000 patients who will constitute the active patient population of the network of community health centers.

Periodic interrogation of the data base has yielded useful information on the prevalence of health problems seen in the center over a period of time (Figure 5).

Problem	Number of Encounters	Frequency
Upper respiratory infection	212	8.0%
Hypertension/hypertensive cardiovasc. dis.	165	6.2%
Obesity	138	5.2%
Diabetes mellitus	114	4.3%
Pregnancy	76	2.9%
Otitis media	72	2.7%
Degenerative arthritis/joint disease	60	2.3%
Pain or ache (any site)	59	2.2%
Viral infection (unspecified site)	56	2.1%
Miscellaneous mental/emotional problem	56	2.1%
Laryngitis/pharyngitis	54	2.0%
Accident/injury	53	2.0%
Tuberculosis	52	2.0%
Socio-economic problem	50	1.9%
Poor vision/blurred vision	49	1.8%
Anxiety	46	1.7%
Coronary artery disease	42	1.6%
Miscellaneous dermatologic problem	38	1.4%
Urinary tract infection	38	1.4%
Miscellaneous eye problem	37	1.4%
Dermatides	36	1.4%
Tonsillitis/adenoiditis	34	1.3%
Pediculosis and other skin parasites	31	1.2%
Pneumonia/pneumonitis	31	1.2%
Vaginitis (all forms)	29	1.1%
Impetigo/erysipelas/pyodermia	28	1.1%
Bronchitis, not chronic	27	1.0%
Constipation	26	1.0%
Gastroenteritis/gastritis/enteritis	26	1.0%
Depression/depressive reaction	26	1.0%

Fig. 5: Problem Profile (January 1976).

Encounters for Most Frequently Named Problems or Diagnoses

Also statistical summaries of the volume of services rendered at
each center are provided (Figure 6) as well as a report of the
socio-demographic characteristics of the active users (Figure 7).

HARRIS COUNTY HOSPITAL DISTRICT
CASA DE AMIGOS NEIGHBORHOOD CLINIC
DEMOGRAPHIC REPORTS
01/01/77 THROUGH 03/31/77

*** PATTERNS OF UTILIZATION ***

	FEMALE		MALE		TOTAL	
SERVICES + ENCOUNTERS	PATIENTS	VISITS	PATIENTS	VISITS	PATIENTS	VISITS
M. D. PROVIDER	2634	6230	1234	2782	3868	9012
M. P. S.	159	454	73	140	232	504
NURSE	3573	21451	1569	3553	5142	25004
LABORATORY	1420	3204	485	1120	1905	4324
RX REFILL	2409	5635	1156	2644	3565	8279
EYE MOBILE	150	380	80	175	230	555
SOCIAL WORKER	107	410	52	150	159	560
NUTRITIONIST	314	1631	102	257	416	1888
MENTAL HEALTH	31	83	9	32	40	115
ELIGIBILITY INT.	925	2378	540	1209	1465	3587
HOME VISIT	30	106	14	44	44	150
HOSPITAL VISIT	8	23	1	1	9	24
M. H. - M. R.	121	985	108	294	229	1279
DENTIST	15	46	4	10	19	56
RADIOLOGY	421	960	209	483	630	1443
HEALTH EDUC.	80	205	31	89	111	294
MEDICAL INFO.	1	1			1	1
OTHER	356	945	127	314	483	1259
TOTALS	12754	45127	5794	13297	18548	58424

Fig. 6: Casa de Amigos Neighborhood Clinic.
Demographic Report

*** SOCIO-ECONOMIC PATTERNS ***

	FEMALE		MALE		TOTAL	
	PATIENTS	VISITS	PATIENTS	VISITS	PATIENTS	VISIT
GROUP						
NEGRO	106	134	33	48	139	182
WHITE	42	55	22	29	64	84
SPANISH ORIGIN	311	398	156	192	467	5n0
ORIENTAL	11	14	2	2	13	16
OTHER	4	5	4	5	8	10
SEX						
KNOWN	475	607	217	276	692	883
UNKNOWN					1	1
AGE						
UNDER 1 YEARS	9	14	18	22	30	39
1-5 YEARS	33	43	30	34	71	85
6-10 YEARS	21	27	26	30	46	59
11-15 YEARS	29	33	23	27	52	57
16-20 YEARS	31	37	6	6	37	43
21-30 YEARS	70	85	10	12	84	1n5
31-40 YEARS	52	74	11	12	60	81
41-50 YEARS	60	70	17	22	73	86
51-60 YEARS	80	108	24	36	108	151
61-65 YEARS	36	46	13	20	49	65
66 + YEARS	52	68	38	54	83	113
NOT AVAILABLE	2	2	1	1		
EDUCATION						
4TH GRADE OR LESS	177	228	131	163	309	302
5TH-8TH GRADE	135	183	41	50	176	233
9TH-12TH GRADE	81	99	25	33	106	132
HIGH SCHOOL GRAD	44	51	11	17	55	68
NOT AVAILABLE	26	31	9	13	35	44
EMPLOYMENT						
UNEMPLOYED	186	247	17	21	203	268
EMPLOYED	74	90	28	38	102	128
ON PUBLIC ASSIST	38	50	6	8	44	58
DISABLED	16	17	20	22	36	39
RETIRED	56	72	44	66	100	138
STUDENT	49	55	46	56	95	111
OTHER	54	74	54	62	109	137
NOT AVAILABLE	2	2	2	3	4	5
FAMILY INCOME						
ABOVE POVERTY LINE	89	114	51	63	140	177
BELOW POVERTY LINE	385	492	166	213	552	7n6
HEADS OF FAMILY						
MALE			376	487	376	487
FEMALE	314	394			314	3n4
NOT AVAILABLE					3	3
MARITAL STATUS						
SINGLE	174	211	123	141	298	353
MARRIED	170	227	69	102	239	329
DIVORCED/SEPARATED	51	62	14	17	65	79
WIDOWED	76	100	11	16	87	116
NOT AVAILABLE	4	7				
TOTALS					693	884

Fig. 7: Casa de Amigos Neighborhood Clinic.
Socio-economic patterns report

The data base has been interrogated frequently for specific research purposes as well as for periodic assessments of care quality. From an education standpoint, the computerized summary documents have been of great usefulness in the teaching of medical students and students of allied health professions who rotate through the centers for training in the management of primary care problems.

Computer Simulation Studies

Gorry and coworkers ( ) have used the data collected on the delivery of emergency medical services in Houston to construct a mathematical model which predicts the performance of a community-wide emergency medical system as a function of the number of its ambulances. The model predicts the probability that a given emergency will be served within a given time interval from the time an ambulance is dispatched to the scene of the emergency. Figure 8 shows the computed probabilities of timely interventions within three specified time intervals of 5, 10 and 15 minutes.

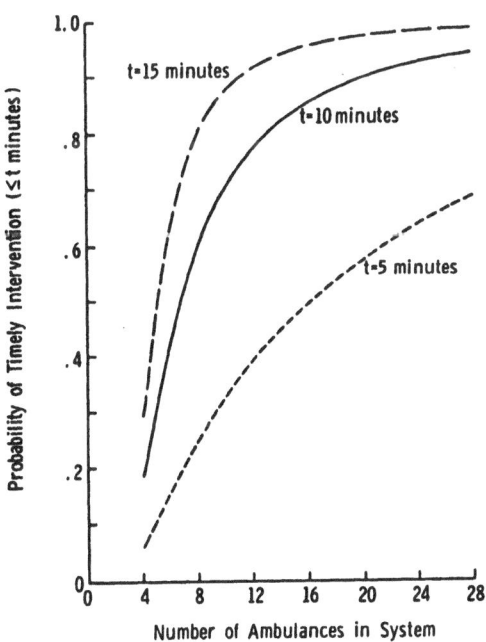

Fig. 8: Probabilities of timely interventions within three specified time intervals

Gorry and Scott ( ) have also developed a model to analyze the cost-effectiveness of training large numbers of citizens in the techniques of cardiopulmonary resuscitation. The model considers as key factors the maximum distance from which a person who has previously trained might be able to intervene in an emergency, the cost of training, and the potential loss of skill with time. Figure 9 shows an analysis generated by the model on the cost that

Retraining interval (T) and cost in dollars per trainee (c)	Total cost per year in dollars	Fraction of population trained in CPR
CRITICAL DISTANCE = 1500 FT		
12-month retraining interval		
$5 per trainee	17 000	1/352
$10 per trainee	34 000	1/352
6-month retraining interval		
$5 per trainee	34 000	1/176
$10 per trainee	68 000	1/176
CRITICAL DISTANCE = 500 FT		
12-month retraining interval		
$5 per trainee	153 000	1/39
$10 per trainee	307 000	1/39
6-month retraining interval		
$5 per trainee	307 000	1/19.5
$10 per trainee	614 000	1/19.5
CRITICAL DISTANCE = 250 FT		
12-month retraining interval		
$5 per trainee	614 000	1/9.8
$10 per trainee	1 228 000	1/9.8
6-month retraining period		
$5 per trainee	1 228 000	1/4.9
$10 per trainee	2 456 000	1/4.9

Fig. 9: Cost for Houston, Texas, to achieve an expected effectiveness of 90 percent

would be incurred in Houston to achieve an expected effectiveness of 90% of a community-wide program of training in cardiopulmonary resuscitation.

These two examples are presented to emphasize the value of simulation technology in community health planning. Theoretical projections of cost can be made if health services researchers have ready access to data bases that contain accurate information on the volume of health services rendered to a given population and on the prevalence of health problems in that community.

Acceptance of Technology

A question frequently posed by health professionals is the extent
to which low income persons accept new technology. In our experience,
technological developments have been very well accepted by the users
of the community health centers. In 1973, before we began the
development of a computerized ambulatory information system,
Spencer and coworkers ( ) conducted a study of the attitudes and
expectations of community residents who had been thoroughly
informed about the scope of our project. Their attitudes were
contrasted to those of the research staff responsible for the
development of the system and with those of the professional and
administrative personnel of the center. Figure 10 showshow positive
attitudes were articulated by the consumer council of patients.

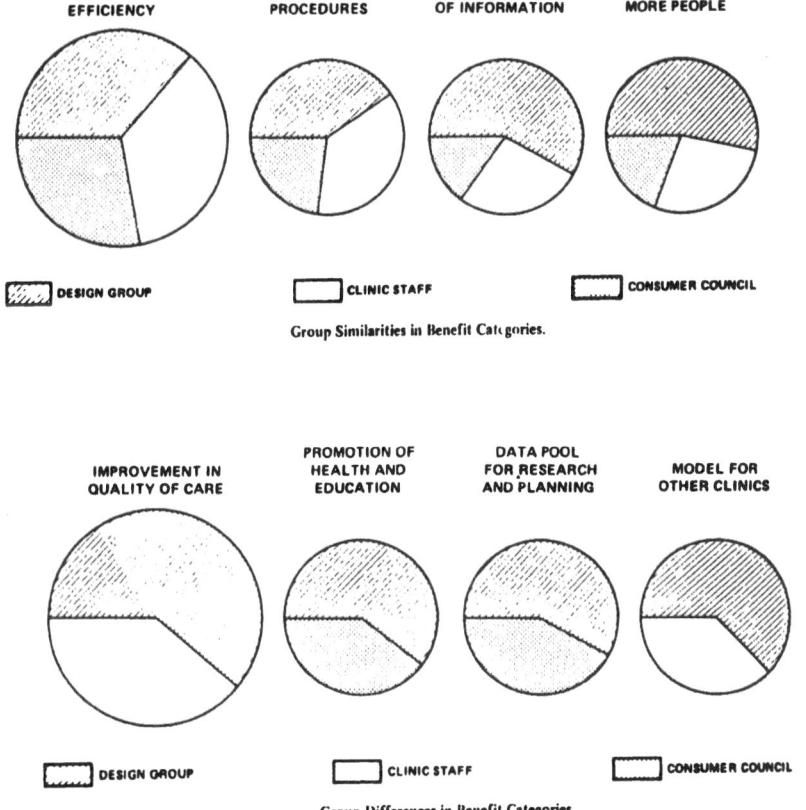

Fig. 10: Group similarities and differences in
benefit categories

After the system had been in operation for one year, <u>Beggs-Baker</u>
and coworkers ( ) conducted a detailed study of attitudes of health
professionals, administrative staff, and consumers. The study
pointed out the high degree of acceptance on the part of all groups
and at no point did we encounter problems of unauthorized access
to confidential data.

A Health Care Information System for Regional Planning in Transition from a Centralized to a Distributed System

H. Peterson

Stockholm County has a population of about 1.5 million. The Stockholm County Council Medical Services Board has under its jurisdiction 71 hospitals with a total of 20,700 beds. The total number of out-patient visits handled by the 1,450 county employed physicians is about 3.7 million per year. Of these physicians 350 are employed as district physicians out in the field and 1,100 at the different hospitals.

To help handle the flow of information between individual physicians, medical departments and hospitals, a regional information system for health care planning has been developed (Figure 1).

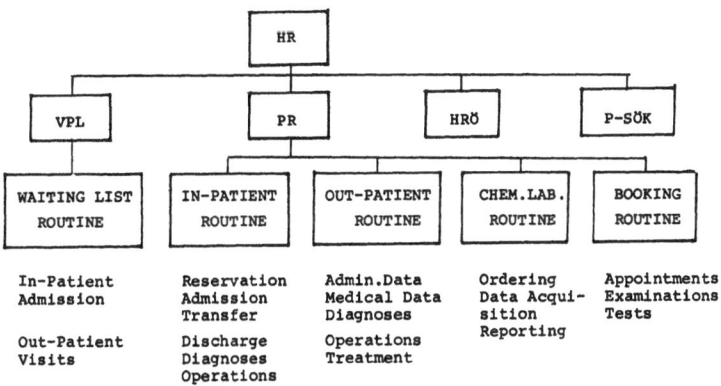

HR = Master Index   PR = Patient File   VPL = Waiting List Routine
HRÖ = Patient Identity Information   P-SÖK = Identity Number Search

Fig. 1: Stockholm County Information System for Health Care Planning

At present the system serves 18 hospitals where a total of 320
terminals are installed.

Regional Information System for Health Care Planning

The Master Index is on-line and represents one of the basic functions
of the information system. This file comprises relevant basic data
on all presumptive patients, that means all inhabitants of the
county.

The file contains:

(1) Census information (official personal data, address etc.)
     (The file is updated every week by means of
      magnetic tapes from the Central Population Registry.),

(2) Vital medical information,

(3) Information on previous in-patient care,

(4) Information on previous x-ray examinations.

The information in (2)-(4) above is built up from a number of
modules, each containing information on the treatment of the patient,
making it possible to follow the patient from the initial contact
with the hospital to the end of the treatment in out-patient as
well as in-patient care. The index information on previous in-
patient care and x-ray examinations is available from 1969 onwards.

For current patients, a special Patient File for each hospital or a
group of hospitals has been created. This file is on direct access
memory, but information is only stored during the time that the
person is actually a patient. After that period the information is
partly transferred to the Master Index and partly to the Medical
History File. This file is stored on magnetic tape.

Medical Statistics

As the Master Index contains vital statistical data for the entire
population of the county together with the medical data, many
different statistics can be produced.

The records of departed persons are transferred from the Master
Index to a special file kept only for statistical reasons. On the

same file are also stored all changes in the vital statistical data.
Thus it is possible to make studies on the population as it was
at any previous time.

Certain statistical reports are produced regularly, in particular

- operational, showing the number of patients and length of
  stay for all diagnoses or groups of diagnoses or any types
  of surgery for different departments, hospitals and the
  entire county. These reports are produced every 6 months,
  covering half a year and one year periods and divided by
  age and sex.

- operational, showing the breakdown of diagnoses for different
  parts of the county and divided by age and sex. Produced
  only for requested diagnoses.

- individual follow-up or selective clinical research to
  include any part or parts of the information stored, and
  sorted in any desired way. These are produced on request
  on a day-to-day basis, mostly for individual physicians.

  (At the moment this possibility is used approximately 50 times
  per month and is very much appreciated.)

- operational, showing the distribution of costs of tests and
  examinations to the referring unit, using a point system.

Use of the Information System for Health Care Planning

The planning process in the Stockholm County contains three levels

- Development plan,
- Operational plan,
- 1 - 5 year budget.

The above mentioned medical statistics are used as a basis for all
three planning instruments. In addition to this, a number of special
studies are performed such as

- The geographical distribution of care consumption,
- Estimates of care consumption,
- Changing trends in the panorama of diseases,
- Measuring the demand for medical care.

The Geographical Distribution of Care Consumption

Within Stockholm County, an area of approx. 6,500 square kilometres, there is a large number of medical and health care institutions and hospitals. There are 13 hospitals for acute somatic care. The total number of clinics amounts to about 200.

In order to establish an acceptable allocation of resources and an even distribution of the work load at the institutions, all these units/clinics have been assigned a geographical catchment area from which patients are recruited. The ultimate intention of this system is that all patients, regardless of the nature of their ailment, should have an equally good opportunity of obtaining health and medical care services.

Not many years ago, a data base project was initiated in order to survey the geographic distribution of the consumption of medical care. This survey now gives annual information on the distribution of consumption of medical care.

In summary, it can be said that this information is produced by simultaneous processing of the diagnostic data mentioned earlier, containing a record of 250,000 - 300,000 hospitalisation cases annually and a population data file on every person resident in the county during the year. When compared with the manual bed-occupancy statistics, the shortfall in the diagnosed in-patient cases has been less than 5% throughout.

There are possibilities for obtaining a variety of data tables in accordance with the planning question to be dealt with. The material has been standardised for age groups so that the varying age distribution in the 160 parishes of the county, with its 23 municipal districts and 13 basic recruiting or catchment areas, does not affect the relative figures obtained for care consumption.

One of the tables gives a breakdown of the care consumed in Stockholm County in terms of 20 age groupings of five years each, and in terms of male and female. For each of these age group categories the actual medical care consumed can be read in terms of bed-days, number of patients and number of admissions. Furthermore, the population in each age group is indicated. The quotients for relating care consumed to the number of inhabitants are also stated. This basic table is presented for three different diagnosis levels as well as in the form of several special data runs, for example for somatic acute care and psychiatry.

Another table called Comparative Use or Consumption indicates the actual, the expected and the age-standardised consumption of care for each parish and municipal district in the county. Bed-days, number of patients and admissions constitute the basis of description here as well. The number of inhabitants per parish and municipal district is also indicated together with certain quotients which enable direct comparisons to be made of the relative care consumption in different geographical areas. An expected use or consumption of 100 corresponds to the average for the county as a whole. Here,too, three levels of diagnoses are technically possible.

A third type of table presents the actual and expected use per age group and parish.   The factors described are basically the same as before. Actually, the only innovation is the age classification. Any group of diagnoses or any level of diagnosis is technically feasible.

A few of these basic tables are of special interest from the point of view of medical care planning.

With a table on comparative use or consumption of medical care it is possible to compare the relative use of hospital care within various recruiting or catchment areas (or for some other geographical distribution).

Use or consumption is measured in terms of the number of patients. The index 100 indicates the "normal" use of medical care for the county as a whole. The material is indirectly standardised for age groupings and covers all admissions for in-patient care in the county.

The results indicate that there are considerable variations in the amount of hospitalisation consumed. These variations can be interpreted in at least two ways. The variations may reflect an actual difference in the need for medical care and/or a demand for medical care that is conditioned by socio-economic factors. Another interpretation could be that differences in the organisational structure of medical facilities account for variations in use. Since in this case the material is derived from in-patient hospital care, it can be assumed that, as a rule, the variations reflect the first mentioned explanation even if it has not yet been proven statistically. The

fact that variations arise within one and the same recruiting area
also speaks in favour of that conclusion.

Estimates of Care Consumption

The data base information system is already being used in order to
seek to equalize the patient burden at the various hospitals and also
to dimension bed capacity within the field of the basic disciplines.
This is achieved by means of consumption estimates for the basic
recruiting areas. The starting point of the calculations is the
number of bed-days per five year group during a given year within
the county area as a whole. The series of figures obtained for 20
five year groups is applied to the population within the respective
basic recruiting area. Adding the figures for all the age groups
produces a total figure - a consumption figure which can be determined
for each individual basic recruiting area.

The method thus makes it possible to take age structure into
consideration when destributing resources and thus not only the
absolute size of the population.

Changing Trends in the Panorama of Diseases

The statistics on health and medical care which have been presented
in the foregoing have been available in data base form since 1971.
They constitute an excellent basis for studying various types of
long-term changes within and outside the medical care organisation.

The long-term changes in the panorama of diseases constitute a
decisive factor which must provide a basis for any long-term planning
in health and medical care.

The individual-based diagnostic statistics form a good starting
point for a description of how different diagnoses co-variate with
age, sex and residential districts in the county area. In our county
specialised knowledge of the significance of age in this connection
has been of great value and has justified a major expansion of
somatic long-term care, while taking account of the special pattern
of diagnoses in that branch of care.

Current statistics also make it possible to study the effects of
different types of preventive measures. An example of this is the
decrease in some children's diseases which is verifiable and which
is related to the expansion of the child health care programme.

It is most important, in the prevailing situation, to concentrate on following up those diagnoses groups whose development is related to certain aspects of the development of society. This applies to damage from alcohol, smoking and narcotics and the consequences of environmental pollution in its various forms. Various states of psychological stress should also be studied. This type of follow-up is presented in the annual statistical reports which are published by the Health and Medical Service Board of the County Council.

Measuring the Demand for Medical Care

A fundamental principle of medical care planning in Stockholm is to make clear distinctions between different forms of care so that a structure can be obtained that permits rational exploitation of resources.

The principle of distinct forms of care implies that the methods of analysis will be different for the different forms of care.

In the most recent long-term planning for that form of care, a model has been applied which in the first instance is designed to select the categories of patients who could be cared for equally well in long-term care rather than acute somatic care. The criteria for what can be regarded as acute care have been set at a maximum of 30 days care. Empirical study has shown that the hypothesis of 30 days, as a limiting value for adequately dimensioning acute care, is reasonably generous. Actual conditions suggest that the limit could probably be set much lower.

The basic statistical material upon which the dimensioning of somatic acute care is founded consists of facts on all the patients that have been discharged during one year. The patient statistics have been compiled for age groups of five year intervals in order to correspond to the comparable descriptions of the population prognoses.

The analysis of demand starts with the number of in-patients and then proceeds by comparing the patients in the different age groups with the population in the same age groups in the county area. A figure is thereby obtained for the proportion of care recipients as a percentage of the population. Assuming no change in the frequency of disease in the different age groups, the currently derived care percentages can be applied to the future population. By this the quantity or expected number of patients ten to fifteen years ahead can be predicted.

In order to further estimate the future number of beds required, assumptions must be made about the average number of bed-days in the future and the bed occupancy rate.

The information stored is also available for other studies using special programs.

There now exists the unique possibility to follow the morbidity of a population of 1.5 million inhabitants on an individual basis.

The content of the Master Index will be increased to contain vital medical information from tests and examinations. Together with this the statistical programs will be revised so that trend analyses covering many years can be obtained. Integrated statistics and prognostications are under development, e.g. distribution and economic results on treatment of different diagnoses from in- and out-patient care and their effect, e.g. number of doctors and other resources to be employed at different treatment levels. The final aim should, of course, be to aid the long-range planning of medical care under all aspects, e.g. buildings and personnel, hospital and home care, transportation and administration.

The philosophy for the system can be expressed as follows:

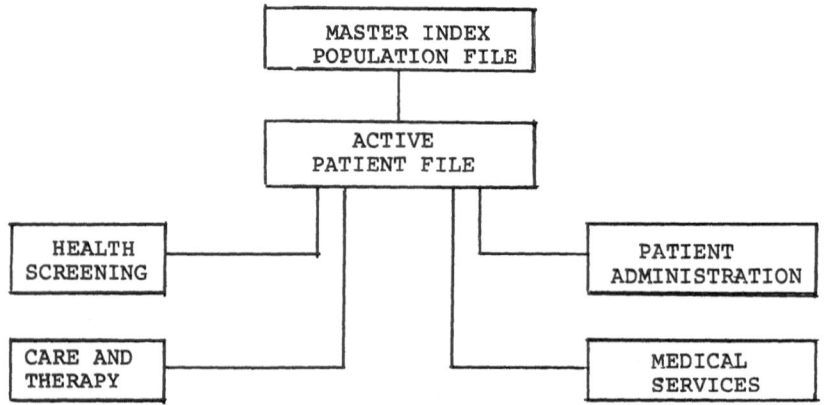

The system structure can functionally be divided into the
following levels:

- Central function for a region including Master Index,
  Health Screening and Statistics,

- Local functions for each hospital or groups of hospitals,
  including Active Patient Files, Patient Administration
  and parts of Care and Therapy,

- Peripheral functions for specific laboratories and
  departments including Medical Services and part of
  Care and Therapy.

Transition from a Centralized to a Distributed System

This philosophy and system structure is used in our centralized
system and will not be changed in our distributed system under
development. Computers linked together in a network will be used
on each level of the structure to handle the functions mentioned.

References

1. Fenna, D., Abrahamsson, S. Lööw, S.O., Peterson, H.:
   The Stockholm County Medical Information System. Lecture Notes
   in Medical Informatics, Vol. 2 (Berlin-Heidelberg-New York:
   Springer, 1978).

2. Peterson, H., Fenna, D.: Medical informatics and privacy
   legislation in Sweden. Biosci. Comm. 2 (1978) 306-312.

3. Undall, B., Kogeus, K., Lindelöw, B., Manson, G., Peterson, H.
   Pettersson, L.: Simplified methods for evaluation of health care
   information systems, currently used by Stockholm County.
   In D.B. Shires, H. Wolf (Eds.): MEDINFO 77. Proceed. Second
   World Conf. Med. Informat., pp. 917-921. (Amsterdam-New York-
   Oxford: North-Holland Publ. Co. 1977).

Health Information System and Health Reform in Italy

A. Serio

Introduction

Law No. 833 introduced for the first time in Italy a set of
provisions expressly devoted to the Health Information System (HIS).

Some of these provisions are finalized to prevent activities to be
implemented at the Local Health Unit (LHU) level. Of major
importance among them is the determination of data on the "factors
of harmfulness, dangerousness and deterioration of living and
working environments" (article 20, a), and the drawing up of
"risk maps" to reveal the noxious substances of industrial origin,
and their possible effects on man and on the environment
(article 20, d).

Of a really innovative content are the provisions relating to the
"communication of the data obtained" and to the "spreading of the
knowledge" within the places of work and throughout the LHU
territory (article 20, b), insofar as these provisions introduce
for the first time the obligation to circulate health information
outside the sphere of those who operate in the health field
(experts, managers, persons in charge of services, etc.) in order
to ensure the participation of the user in the knowledge of
problems and, hence, in the operation of services.

The same law also defined the information tools to be used by the
National Health Service and indicated them in the personal health
card and in the biostatistical data registers (article 27); the
former obviously represents an individual information tool whose
aim is essentially auxiliary in that it allows each health
operator, with whom the user comes into contact, to learn any
information on the latter's state of health; the registers

containing biostatistical environmental data represent, instead, information tools chiefly destined for the use of workers.

The same article identifies in the Ministry of Health, in the Regional Authorities and in the Local Health Units as well as in the Higher Institute of Health the bodies entrusted with the task of processing and using the epidemiological data obtained.

Finally, article 58 declares that the activity programs for the determination and handling of all epidemiological information, both statistical and financial, be included in the National Health Plan, and that the Regional Authorities provide for the information services.

Summing up, from the provisions included in the reform law the following guidelines with regard to the subject that interest us emerge:

- Planning is to be viewed as a method for operating the new Health System;

- the availability of adequate health information is essential for the purposes of planning;

- the health information system is the tool to be set in motion in order to ensure the availability of the data required.

Objectives of the Information System

The Health Information System (HIS) consists of the instruments, the personnel and the procedures taken as a whole that are required for the acquisition and processing of the data useful for the following purposes:

- knowledge of the health conditions of the population;

- health planning;

- health services management.

Organization of Information Systems

HIS has to be organized taking into account the particular
features of the health services, the nature of the information to
be handled, and the way the National Health Service is organized.
Various territorial levels are thus to be envisaged, with varying
functions and characteristics.

1) At the district level, the survey of the data concerning the
   residing citizens is to be envisaged;no processing activity - for
   which a number of resources is required that are only available
   at higher territorial levels - is foreseen.

2) At the LHU level, the survey of data which refer to the health
   services operating in the territory of competence is envisaged;
   also envisaged is filing and processing all data - wherever
   determined - that refer to the population usually present in the
   territory. This involves the realization of the Local
   Information System (LIS), being the field operational unit of the
   Health Information System.

   It receives and provides information to the following services
   operating in the territory:

   - health services proper;

   - other social and health services (day nurseries, schools,
     factories, old peoples' homes, etc.);

   - administrative services for the management of health
     structures;

   - other information systems (municipal register offices,
     etc.).

   The health services proper include:

   - background services (general practitioners, paediatric
     medicine, public health services, etc.);

   - intermediate services (special out-patients' departments);

   - hospital services.

LIS is organized according to modular criteria, taking into account
the resources and features of the territory. In the large cities,
an intermediate level or district is to be envisaged, which includes
more than one LHU and which takes up the duties of the relevant
information systems.

3) The Regional Information System (RIS) represents the place
where all health information concerning the region is
collected and processed; no survey of individual data is
foreseen at this level.

RIS supervises the health situation and the activity of the
services of the various LHUs; it processes the data needed for
regional health planning and for the epidemiological observation
post;it conveys to the National Information System the
information required for National Health Planning.

Information to be Obtained and Processed

The information items to be collected and processed are divided
into individual data (referring to individuals) and collective
data (referring to services and structures). The latter may be
further divided into:

- environmental data,

- population and social data,

- data on the activity of health services,

- data of health interest obtained from other sources.

Individual health data include the principal information items
determined on the occasion of the contacts between each citizen and
the health structures; events that are often conducive to a contact
with the Service are the following:

- pregnancies, either normal or with complications,

- pathological or physiological deliveries,

- psycho-physical development,

- vaccinations,

- cases of sickness,

- cases of accidents (occupational or non-occupational),

- cases of permanent or temporary disability.

Also to be envisaged are surveys of some basic clinical
informative items that are useful chiefly in cases of emergency
(blood group, serious chronic diseases, allergies and intolerance
to particular drugs, etc.) which, taken as a whole, may be defined
as "clinical background history".

Environmental data refer to the conditions of soil, of water, of the atmosphere, and concern both the territory in general and specific environments (places of work, school communities, etc.).

Population and social data include the main information items on each individual and on the entire population (personal data and economic and social data).

Data on the activity of health services include all information on personnel, on equipment and on the services rendered by hospital and non-hospital services.

Finally data will be included that, although obtained from other sources (municipal register offices, censuses, manpower surveys, etc. ...), are of interest from the point of view of health.

Standardization of the Data Survey Methods

It will be clear from the foregoing that, following the implementation of the health reform, in-depth modifications will be made in the survey of health data, a task that has been carried out so far by the national bodies and that is now entrusted to the local health units and to the regional authorities. The necessity thus arises to ensure at the national level the standardization of the methods used for obtaining the data in order to guarantee the comparability of the data emerging from the various areas of the Italian territory and from other countries.

For this purpose, one of the first objectives to be attained is the identification of the information items that are deemed essential for the knowledge about the health conditions of the population and for health planning.

The necessity of making reference - as far as the data on the causes of death, on the cases of illness and on hospitalizations are concerned - to the International Classification of Diseases (9th Revision) being beyond doubt, the convenience ought to be examined of utilizing, in relation to specific types of data, reduced classifications already drawn up on the basis of the special survey requirements. Similar problems are indicated with regard to the data on the activities of the health services for which an "ad hoc" classification was recently developed by WHO.

In coping with this set of problems, account should be taken of the convenience of formulating social and health indicators suited for assessing the health conditions of the population and the efficiency of the health services, also in relation to the resources employed.

Health of a Region - Example: Ontario, Canada

D.J. Shepley

Introduction

Canada is a nation of approximately 25 million people settled in ten provinces and two territories. The provinces range in population from just over 100,000 in Prince Edward Island to approximately eight million in Ontario. Three levels of government exist with a fourth emerging. These include the federal, the provincial, the emerging regional level and the municipal governments.

The provision of health care is primarily a provincial responsibility. I will be reviewing our health scene as I find it as a general practitioner in Ontario.

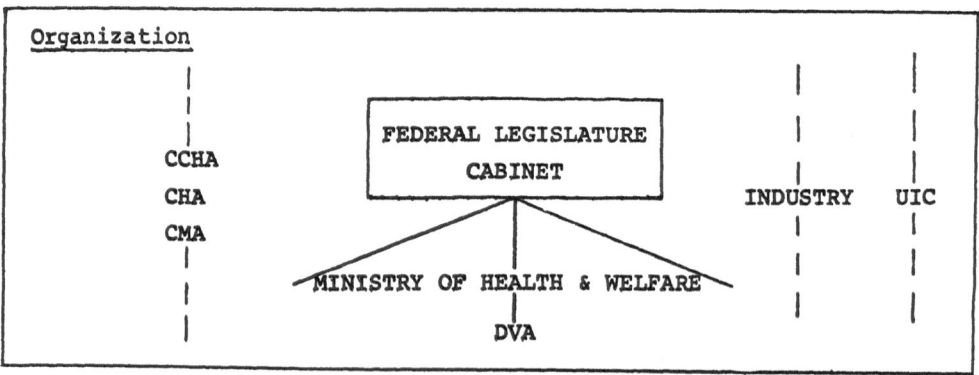

Fig. 1: Federal Relationships (CCHA = Canadian Council for Hospital Accreditation, CHA = Canadian Hospital Association, CMA = Canadian Medical Association, DVA = Department of Veterans Affairs, UIC = Unemployment Insurance Commission)

Figure 1 outlines very briefly the structure, organization and
relationship among the government health-related bodies, for example,
the legislature with its cabinet, one of the major ministries (the
Ministry of Health and Welfare), professional organizations, for
example, The Canadian Hospital Association (CHA), The Canadian
Medical Association (CMA), The Canadian Council on Hospital
Accreditation (CCHA), and other non-government agencies (embodied
in the term "industry"). The UIC (Unemployment Insurance Commission)
is a semi-governmental agency reporting directly to the Legislature.

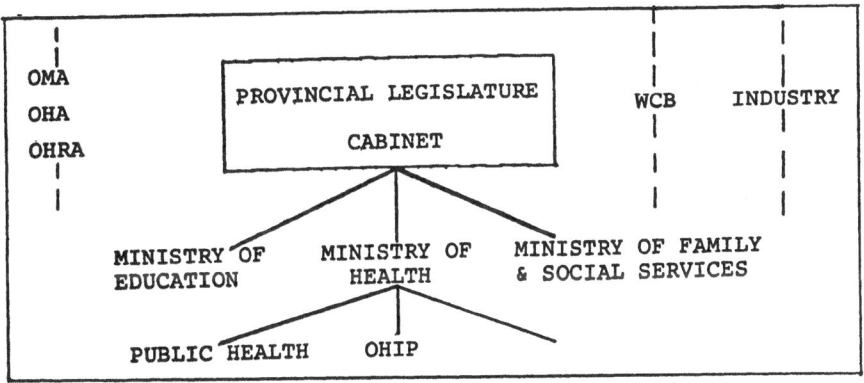

Fig. 2: Provincial Relationships (OMA = Ontario Medical Association,
        OHA = Ontario Hospital Association, OHRA = Ontario Hospital
        Records Association, WCB = Workmen's Compensation Board,
        OHIP = Ontario Health Insurance Plan)

You will note an almost identical structure in Figure 2. Here in
Ontario, however, Health and Family and Social Services (welfare)
are separate ministries. The professional bodies parallel, to some
extent, the national bodies. As in Figure 1, other non-governmental
bodies are represented as "industry". The Workmen's Compensation
Board (WCB) is a provincial body reporting to the Legislature.

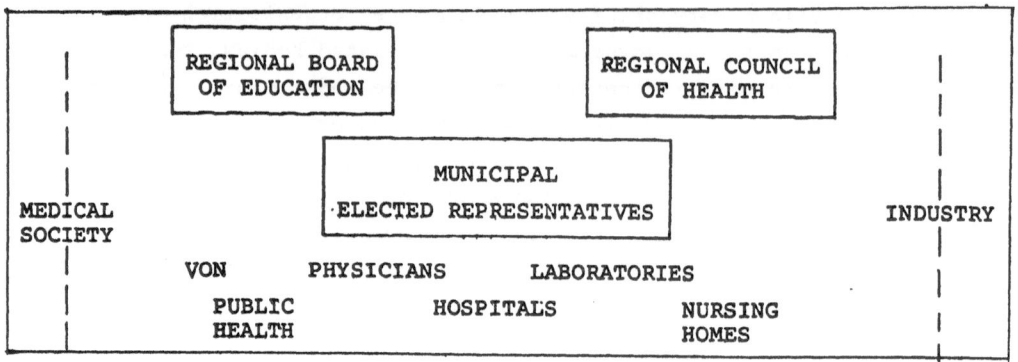

<u>Fig. 3</u>: Municipal Relationships (VON = Victorian Order of Nurses)

Figure 3 again parallels the structure outlined in Figure 1;
however, the actual agencies providing health care services are
shown as well. These include hospitals, laboratories, and
physicians.

The significant development in our area is the emerging fourth
level of government represented here by the regional entities: The
Regional Board of Education and The Regional Council of Health.
In the area where I live and practice, The Durham Regional Council
of Health has just been struck. Its function at this point is
primarily advisory to the Ministry of Health.

Several key concepts are responsible for this organization and the
inter-relationships. I believe one of the most significant factors
has been the ability to fund or render payment on a massive scale,
particularly through the use of computer-based insurance systems.
Because of this, other factors have become significant.

Centralization

In order to effect some equalization of health care costs across
Canada, the Federal Government adopted the concept of "universality".
This meant that "all people" in "all provinces" would be covered
for "all services". The Federal Government induced the provincial
governments to adopt this approach through its cost-sharing programs.

In order to participate, the provinces had to show that 98% of the population was covered for "all services".

In that most of the private insuring bodies did not cover "all services", the insuring body became an arm of the provincial government. In Ontario it became the Ontario Health Insurance Plan (OHIP).

Decentralization

It soon became apparent, however, that there was a limit to funds. The Federal Government first introduced a "limited percentage" of funds for health which would be returned to the provinces through this cost-sharing program. Later the Federal Government altered this policy so that there would be no funds identified for health care specifically. This induced the provinces to increase the proportion of provincial tax monies allocated to pay for health care services. Further, in an attempt to identify the proper disposition of funds, Ontario has gone about setting up regional bodies, i.e. the regional Councils of Health, to set priorities for projects and health dollars in that area. A second step in limiting funds was also introduced, that limiting the percentage of payments provided for services and in addition limiting services supported. Some insurance systems have evolved to provide health care insurance for those entities not covered in the provincial plan. As noted above, in Ontario the main insuring body is the Ontario Health Insurance Plan (OHIP) which is administered through the Ministry of Health.

A Few OHIP Statistics

There are 6,000 hospital discharges each day. There is approximately one quarter million claims processed each workday or about 5 million claims per month for some 8 million people. One estimate may be that approximately 3% of the population is receiving some care at any one time. These claims include those submitted by physicians primarily, but also include chiropractors, hypnotherapists, natural hygienists and dentists.

Privacy and Confidentiality

In such a massive system, with more and more information being
centralized, it is not unexpected there would be problems with the
issue of privacy or confidentiality.

In fact, in Ontario this issue has come forth particularly because
health-related data available through the health insurance system
was brought forward for use other than for health care delivery.
Police and politicians have used it. Public concern has resulted in
striking a commission, headed by the Honorable Mr. Justice Horace
Krever of Toronto, to review all legislation administered by the
Minister of Health, to determine whether proper protection is
given to the rights of persons who have received or may receive
health care services, to preserve the confidentiality of information
about them collected under that legislation, to review the legality
of the administrative process and to make recommendations for any
changes of the legislation. This commission is at present
receiving statements and hearings from the various interested
health-related bodies.

Health Care Delivery from the Practice Viewpoint

I practice in Whitby, a city of approximately 28,000 people which
is physically located between Toronto (2,250,000) and Oshawa
(100,000). The catchment area of approximately a 40 mile radius
has over 250,000 people. I have admitting privileges in the
community hospital with some 65 beds (The Dr. J. O. Ruddy General
Hospital), a regional hospital with some 600 beds (The Oshawa
General Hospital) and a teaching hospital with some 800 beds
(St. Michael's Hospital). I practice within the Ontario Health
Insurance Plan, that is I bill OHIP for services rendered. It should
be noted that OHIP does not cover all services provided and that
the physicians of Ontario are seeking the ability to "balance bill"
the patient for monies not collected through the insurance system
as well as for services not supported by the insurance system.

Referring again to Figures 1, 2 and 3, I bring to your attention
the fact that I have to deal not only with the Ontario Health
Insurance Plan, but directly with the Workmen's Compensation Board,
Social and Family Services, particularly with regard to the elderly,
indirectly with the Unemployment Insurance Commission, the
Department of Veteran's Affairs, the Department of Transport, the

Department of Education, not to mention industry itself,
particularly the private life insurance companies. In dealing with
these bodies, most information is required for payments to the
patient or our clinic and is handled through computer-based systems.

Hospital Committees

In attempting to cope with restricted budgets, the Oshawa General
Hospital has established a Utilization Review Committee and has
charged it with the responsibility of overviewing the use to which
the beds are put. The key component in this is a computer-based
information system providing data about patients based on their
"expected days' stay". Each day a daily monitor report is made
available to members of the staff who act as monitors. This
report contains the following categories:

- Physician
- Chart-No.
- Name of patient
- Consultant
- Diagnosis or procedure group
- Surgery
- Multiple diagnoses
- Physician's estimate of length of stay
- Statistical, average of diagnostic category
- Actual length of stay.

It should be noted that at best the monitors are very reluctant
volunteers, but when available beds are few and there is a
possibility of cancelling surgery, monitors do review patients in
hospital, especially those who are identified through the system
as overstays. I would stress at this point that it is not the
care that is being rendered that is reviewed, rather it is the
delivery of care. We want to "oil the machinery". Most of our
problems have stemmed from lack of communication either between
physician and consultant or physician and nurses. It is this area
that we are trying to prevent from breaking down.

Resource Planning and Care Analysis

Further, because the hospitals are feeling budget restrictions and
are attempting to use every possible means to maintain service with
a relatively reduced budget, another computer-based information
system is used. This system provides information for both planning
of resource allocation as well as information which can act as
a vehicle for study in review of disease entities. The system is
that offered through the Hospital Medical Records Institute (HMRI),
an agency very similar to PAS (Professional Activity Study) in the
United States. In particular, in our hospital we have worked with
HMRI to structure a vehicle for allowing case review, disease
review or procedure review to be carried out in an effective manner
and to minimize the time demanded of each of the participants in
the study. It became apparent very quickly that in order to have
any effective study, there should be consistency in the data
recorded, particularly in diagnosis and procedures. In order to
ensure this, a system for verifying diagnosis was instituted in the
Oshawa General Hospital. In the system, medical records staff
verify that each diagnosis on discharge or each procedure noted on
discharge passes criteria established by the medical staff. In this
way, some consistency of data is assured. Of course, the criteria
themselves must be reviewed and updated periodically.

Pre-Hospital Cardiac Care Project

I would like to turn now to a more clinically orientated project,
the Pre-Hospital Cardiac Care Project,and draw your attention to
the problems that introducing a relatively new technological
service presents.

This project is a hospital-based project to allow certified emergency vehicle attendants to administer therapy, including
defribrillation, in the field under the express authorization of
the physician in the emergency. This is not a new concept. It does
use telemetry. It does have several extensive systems already
operating to copy. These systems are, e.g. in Los Angeles,
Baltimore, and in Toronto, the latter based jointly at the Sunny-
brook Hospital and the Hospital for Sick Children. Most of the
problems encountered in this project revolve around communication
and training of staff. For information, this project had to be
brought before the following bodies in the hospital: the Intensive
Care Unit Committee, the Emergency Committee, Ambulatory Care

Committee, the Oshawa Emergency Physicians Association, the
Department of General Practice, the hospital administration, the
Medical Advisory Committee executive, the Medical Advisory itself,
the Hospital Board, non-hospital-based bodies: the College of
Physicians and Surgeons, the Ministry of Health, i.e. its Programs
Branch, as well as the branch responsible for insurance, the
Canadian Medical Protective Association, the Department of Trans-
port and Communications for the channels concerned, the Regional
Council of Health. All of these bodies had to be contacted and the
concept discussed before the project was able to go ahead.

Progress

At this point we have received approval from the Regional Council
of Health and are in the process of detailing the equipment to be
bought, the procedures to be carried out, and the education
required for certification. The Ministry will not be funding this;
the hospital foundation will be providing the necessary funds.

Maintenance of the system must be carried out from funds within the
global budget of the hospital. Although the expected costs are
relatively small, there are many costs not identified, e.g.,
people's time.

Conclusion

I have tried to present a brief sketch of the health care scene in
Ontario as seen from a general practitioner's viewpoint. I would
like to stress that technology has played a significant role in
our system. In particular, computer-based technology has affected
three areas. First, the introduction of computers in the insurance
arena has made it possible for the massive numbers of people to
be insured and the massive numbers of services to be accounted for.
Further, I feel it is because of this technology our centrally
oriented health system structure was able to evolve.

Although I did not dwell particularly on it, certainly the problems
of privacy and confidentiality related to this information are
causing our government to better define its function in the
provision of this service. Second, computer-based information
systems are making a significant impact in the areas where they
provide information for resource planning and health care analysis

study. Third, computer-based information systems are making an impact at the local level - the delivery of care within the hospital itself, i.e. the systems based on the expected days' stay.

Another area of technology, that of bio-telemetry, is being introduced in our area and, I am sure, it will have a significant impact on the care offered in our region.

I would like to stress a concept that I have not outlined particularly above, that is: the systems, the information, the services provided are only as effective as the people who use them. New problems are emerging with these new technologies. I am sure they can be overcome if prudence is used.

A Rational Care Model for Health Care of a Nation

S.R. Garfield

Enhancement of "Quality of Life" is a major objective of enlightened nations and, since good health is basic to that goal, improved medical care holds high level priority in national planning. Today's massive investment in medical care resources is mute testimony to that fact; yet, despite huge expenditures, there is practically universal dissatisfaction with current medical care systems, particularly with impaired access-ability and maldistribution of physician services and excessive costs. There is a prevalent feeling that health benefits gained are minor, in proportion to the great allocation of resources.

Many reasons have been advanced for the relative failure of our medical care systems to satisfy the needs and expectations of nations; however, the basic reason has passed generally unrecognized, namely, a serious mismatch between today's "Sick Care" delivery systems and the demands and needs of populations. This presentation will focus on that mismatch, explain its cause and suggest a solution.

To begin with, let us have a clear look at the traditional medical care delivery system in the USA. The demand for medical care is not a clear-cut binary sickness present/absent situation. Health is a spectrum consisting of well, worried-well, early-sick, and definitively sick states, with people constantly changing from one state to another and with a great many of them concerned and uncertain about their exact location in that spectrum. That uncertainty creates a tremendous potential demand for medical care which in the past was regulated by the fee mechanism of the market place (see Figure 1.).

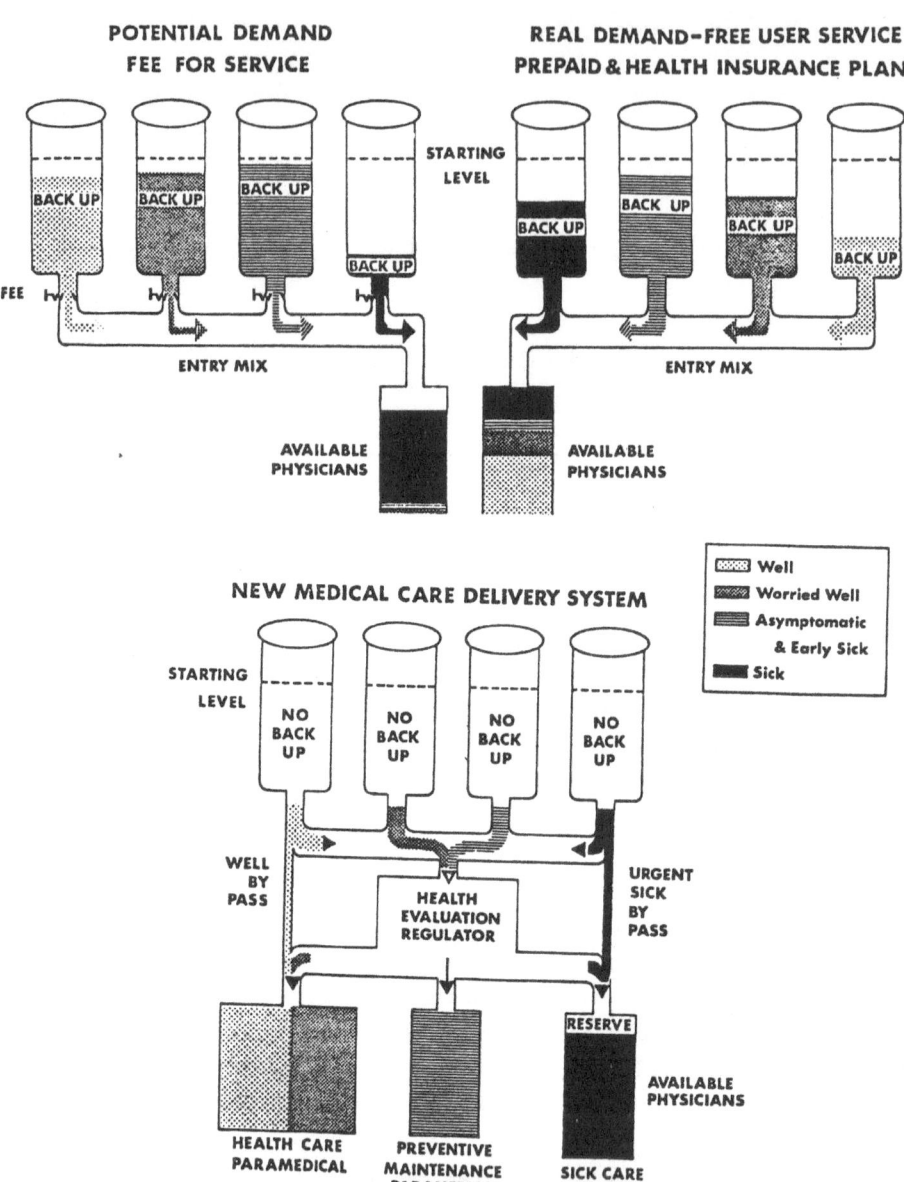

Fig. 1: The traditional medical care delivery system in the USA
and the new concept

With fees, people tend to put off seeing the doctor until definitely sick. They have other uses for their money. This keeps out most of the "uncertainty demand": the well, the worried-well, and the early-sick. Conversely, it admits the definitely sick who seek relief regardless of fee. Thus, fee-for-service demand is predominantly sick demand. The delivery system that has evolved in the USA under two centuries of fee-for-service to match that sick demand is a sick care delivery system with doctors at the point of entry and deeply involved in every step of that sick care process. Likewise, our medical schools have evolved teaching sick care technics. In this sick care system, the fee is the regulator of flow, keeping out "uncertainty demand" and admitting the sick. In general, it is the mechanism that keeps the system demand and supply in balance.

Though the fee is a regulator, it is rather a poor one. There is no real relationship between the need for medical care and ability to pay and the fee does tend to keep out the early sick and quite a few of the sick who cannot afford the cost. In addition, for those who actually enter, the high cost of medical care is very traumatic, so over the years plans have evolved to help the sick: plans such as Blue Cross and Blue Shield, prepaid plans like Kaiser-Permanente, Health Insurance, Medicare and Medicaid, and the many National Health Insurance proposals. All these have one thing in common: They attempt to help the sick secure care by eliminating personally paid fees.

With those facts in mind, let us follow what happens when we eliminate personally paid fees. Our objective, of course, is to guarantee access for the sick who cannot afford today's excessive costs. When we eliminate fees, we lose the regulator of flow into the delivery system. This immediately converts the entire potential "uncertainty demand" into real demand which begins to compete with the sick to get into the delivery system on a first-come, first-served basis. There is no competition from the well under fee-for-service since those people voluntarily stay out of the delivery system. They have other uses for their money. The only real demand under fee-for-service are those who agree to pay and enter the delivery system. Under free care, real demand not only includes those who enter but in addition all those with the slightest wish to enter. They all have an equal right to do so and they become disturbed if they cannot get in for service.

The impact of the tremendous load of uncertainty demand plus the sick
on the delivery system causes four serious problems for medicine:

- It overloads the relatively inelastic sick care delivery system
  causing a backlog of unavailable services; the inevitable queuing
  that goes with free care wherever it has been attempted.

- The large number of well people who actually get into the
  system, by usurping doctor-time, act as a barrier to the entry
  of the sick, the reverse of what we are trying to accomplish by
  eliminating fees.

- With this altered demand, instead of caring for the sick, the
  doctors are spending a large portion of their time trying to
  find something wrong with well people, and they are doing this
  with techniques taught them to diagnose sickness. That reverse
  use of sick care techniques searching for illness in well people
  is extremely wasteful of doctor's time, also irritating and
  frustrating to him.

- The impact of the relatively unlimited amount of "uncertainty
  demand" on the limited supply of physicians inevitably creates
  inflationary costs.

Those are among the most urgent problems facing medicine today, not
only in this country but in many others of the world. They have all
fallen into the same difficulty of eliminating the fee-regulating
mechanism, then trying to funnel the large "uncertainty demand" plus
the sick through the existing sick care system. Not only is this
physically impossible, but "uncertainty demand", with its large
component of well people, is incompatible with direct entry through
sick care physician services; incompatible, because it does not
match the techniques of sick care. Sick care diagnosis is a clue-
directed, step-by-step search for patterns of illness, which can be
performed efficiently by the physician, if the patient is clearly sick
and clues are definite. "Uncertainty demand" has vague, misleading
or absent clues, requiring a different approach. The diagnostic
procedure here becomes a meticulous checking out of all systems, a
comprehensive countdown process that is most efficiently performed
by protocolized paramedical services, not by the doctor. If we do
use doctors for that countdown process, as we are actually doing all
through this country, we get into the incongruous situation of using
up an enormous amount of doctor-time searching for the relatively
few people who need doctor-time, leaving little time available for
the care of the sick. This is a self-defeating, vicious circle

phenomenon that drastically dissipates and wastes medical manpower and is the chief reason for unavailability of services today.

It should be clear that the basic cause of our medical care problem has been the increasing spread of free user care throughout our population. The effect is an expanded and altered demand that is largely incompatible with the existing sick care system, wasting its medical manpower, rendering the system unbalanced and seriously defective. An understanding of this cause and effect relationship leads us to a solution. The existing medical care system, designed to care for the sick, matches only the "sick demand". Balancing the system necessitates that "uncertainty demand" be similarly matched with a suitable service. This requires two changes. The usual way one enters medical care today is through physician services. This is not only wasteful of medical manpower but a serious bottleneck as well. So, first we must provide a new method of entry, other than through the physician; a method which can separate free user demand into its basic components: the well, the asymptomatic sick and the sick. Second, we must provide an adequate service to receive each of these components.

The new method of entry we have developed is "Health Testing". The services are a new Health Care Service for the well, a new Preventive Maintenance Service for the asymptomatic sick and high prevalence chronic conditions, and the existing Sick Care Service reserved for the sick.

The new system thus has four divisions (Figure 2), coordinated by computer services:

1. Health Testing - the heart of the new system combines a detailed automated medical history with comprehensive panels of physiological and laboratory tests administered by paramedical personnel, a physical examination by specially trained nurses and computerized data review and advice rules. Health testing is ideally suited as a new method of entry into medical care since it can effectively separate "uncertainty demand" into its components with a minimum of physician involvement. In addition, it establishes a basic health data base for each individual which becomes the foundation for health or sick care in the future. As such it becomes the basic protocol of medical care.

2. Health Care - is a new division of medicine that does not exist in this country or any country. Its purpose is to improve health and keep people well. To date, health care has been an elusive

142

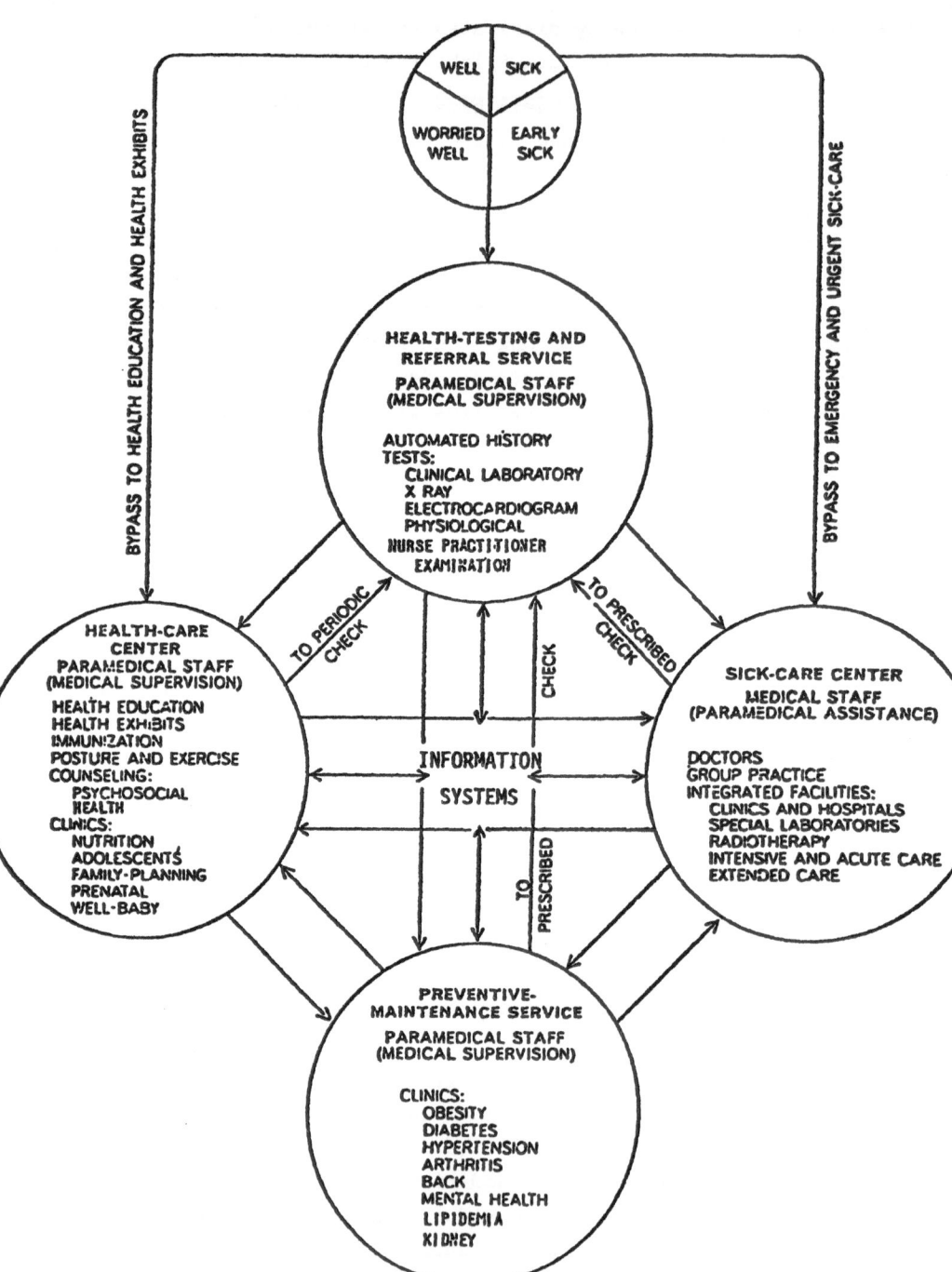

<u>Fig. 2</u>: Schematic representation of new model (modified from
Scientific American 222:4 (April) 1970).

concept, and understandably so, since it has been submerged in sick care, the primary concern of doctors. Doctors trained in sick care have been much too busy to be involved with well people.

This clear delineation of a Health Care Service is a first step in creating a positive program for keeping people well. This service is essential to meet the increasing demand for health care, to begin keeping people well and to keep these people from using up sick care services.

3. Preventive Maintenance - is a service for the asymptomatic sick and for high-prevalence chronic illness such as hypertension and diabetes, conditions that require monitoring and surveillance. This type of care, performed by protocolized paramedical personnel reporting to the patient's doctor, can relieve the physician of many routine visits.

4. Sick Care - with its high level decisions on diagnosis and therapy remains clearly the realm of the physician. Here he becomes the manager of patient care, rather than the man-of-all-work, and is aided in this by the three other divisions.

There are several important features to be emphasized in this new delivery system:

First - it is designed specifically to match the entry mix of free care with appropriate resources. All other existing systems unload the entire free care entry mix into sick care physician services and thus dissipate and waste medical manpower.

Second - three of the four divisions - Health Testing, Health Care, and Preventive Maintenance - use paramedical services of existing types. Therefore, they are relatively easy to staff and relatively inexpensive. The use of paramedical personnel with limited knowledge and skills to relieve the physician of routine and repetitious tasks requires that such tasks be clearly defined and that patient input be structured. The existing delivery system with its unstructured heterogeneous entry mix is almost the exact antithesis of those requirements and, therefore, has never favored the effective and safe use of such personnel. For this reason Health Testing with its clear separation of services, automatically defining tasks and patient structure, becomes the key to paramedical manpower effectiveness. This effectiveness is greatly enhanced by the guidance made possible by protocols, computerized data review and "advice" rules.

Third - this new system requires no basic modification of sick care services. It can function with either solo practice or group practice. All we need do to sick care is remove from it the extraneous portion of the entry mix produced by free care which does not belong there in the first place. Sick care relieved of that considerable load of well, worried well and asymptomatic sick people thus develops a greatly increased capacity for the care of the sick.

Fourth - medicine past and present has been episodic and crisis-oriented with patients entering for spells of sickness and exiting when presumably cured. The new system changes that. Once entered through health testing, the patient remains in the system with appointments to Health Care, Preventive Maintenance or Sick Care and always with a return appointment to Health Testing for an updating profile. In that fashion much of medicine becomes continuous rather than episodic and much of illness a trend rather than a crisis.

Conclusion

It should be clear that national concern for optimizing the health of populations requires more than a high quality sick care system. Achieving that objective in a cost-effective fashion demands rounding out sick care with the services of Health Evaluation, Health Care and Preventive Maintenance.

One can envision a total health care system of the future which will begin with a basic comprehensive health evaluation for each individual. The results of that evaluation will chart each individual's personal pathway through health care resources. Periodic updating health evaluation profiles will monitor the levels of homeostasis of vital body subsystems and significant deviations will trigger computerized warnings and corrective instructions. Health education will alert and advise measures to be taken against individual predictive risks, be they life style, hereditary, environmental or age-sex linked through time.

Acute illnesses will in large part be entered through protocolized paramedical services and be measured and diagnosed against the background of each individual's updated health profile. Such individualized continuing health care would greatly reduce patient uncertainty and would, in large part, replace today's chaotic random entry demand by a smooth regulated use of appropriate resources that would not only be cost-effective but would also optimize the health of each individual through his lifetime and, thus, would be an ideal system for achieving the objective of the best possible health for the citizens of a nation.

Health Care Supported by Technology in Japan

S. Kaihara

Considering the history of the medical use of computers in Japan, it is possible to identify three stages, as shown in Table 1.

Table 1: Three stages of medical information systems development in Japan

	1968	1973	1978
STAGE OF	INDIVIDUAL TRIAL	GOVERNMENT PARTICIPATION	EVALUATION
Characterized by	Gradual increase of hospital on-site computers	Establishment of MEDIS-DC Interhospital systems Regional systems Research & development	Standardization Safety Cost-effectiveness Technology for Japanese culture
Motivation	Reduction of manpower related to insurance claim	Coordination of medical supply through technology	Health planning Domestic culture oriented technology

The first is the "Individual Trial" stage which started in 1968 and lasted for 5 years. The second is the "Government Participation" stage from 1973 which again lasted for 5 years. The third stage is that from 1978 which may be called the "Evaluation" stage. In the first stage, individual hospitals developed hospital information systems independently with the help of the computer industry. The main motivation in this stage was the reduction of manpower in hospitals related to complicated health insurance claiming activities. Naturally, main efforts have been focused on the development of merely administrative systems. However, in this limited field, several successful systems emerged and the number of hospitals with on-site computers increased in these years.

The second stage was opened by the establishment of the Medical Information System Development Center which is known as "MEDIS-DC". This is a non-profit organization subsidized by the Ministry of

Health and Welfare and the Ministry of International Trade and Industry. With the help of a grant from this organization, inter-hospital or regional systems were developed which could not be accomplished by individual hospitals. The main motivation of MEDIS-DC was the coordination of Japanese health care through technology.

The third stage in computer application to health care - the evaluation stage - has just started in Japan. The increase in medical demands as well as in total medical expenditure directed attention to cost-effective health care. Even technologically successful medical information systems are considered to be in need of reinvestigation from the standpoint of cost-effectiveness. Standardization and safety of the systems are more and more under discussion. Attention is also paid to domestic culture-oriented technologies which will be discussed later. This classification is not official, but made by the author personally but, for better understanding, it will be maintained in the following remarks.

As mentioned above, the individual trials stage started in 1968. Before this year, there was only one hospital in our country which tried an application of computer technology in the medical field. This hospital in the northern part of Japan was brave enough to start the trial in the early sixties but, unfortunately, it failed. The main reason was that the complicated process of data input was not accepted by the hospital personnel. No further attempt was made until 1968 when, with the progress of computer technology, a university hospital in Tokyo had another go with a larger on-line Japanese-made computer system. In the present hospital charging system, part of the charge must be paid by patients at each visit. This means that complicated calculations of the charges to patients must be performed every time patients come to the hospital, while the patients are waiting at the cashier's desk. This can only be done by an on-line computer.

After a few years' struggle, the university hospital finally completed an acceptable system. This system only dealt with patient charging business in a very complicated and tedious manner. Nevertheless, the system was considered to be successful because it relieved accounting personnel of part of the burden of insurance claiming business for the hospital. To understand this, it is necessary to become familiar with Japan's health insurance system. Because of the national health insurance system, hospitals can only charge patients with a small part of the fees. The remainder has to

be submitted to the insurance companies in the form of a claim.
They are non-profit organizations composed of multiple bodies with
different policies. Therefore, hospitals have to describe in the
claim form all details of the medical care which the hospital gave
to the patients, such as names of tests, drugs and operations. The
hospital also has to classify the forms according to the policies
of the insurance company. The hospital submits this form at the end
of each month, even if the patient continues to visit the hospital.
As a result, for example, the University of Tokyo Hospital submits
25,000 sheets of forms per month with detailed descriptions concerning
patient care.

Considering this situation, it was natural that computer applications
should start with this insurance and charging system. Any system
which succeeded in reducing the complicated claiming work was
regarded as a successful system. Encouraged by the success, many
hospitals and small clinics started to develop their own hospital
activities systems. The number of hospital on-site computers
increased year after year, as seen in Fig. 1.

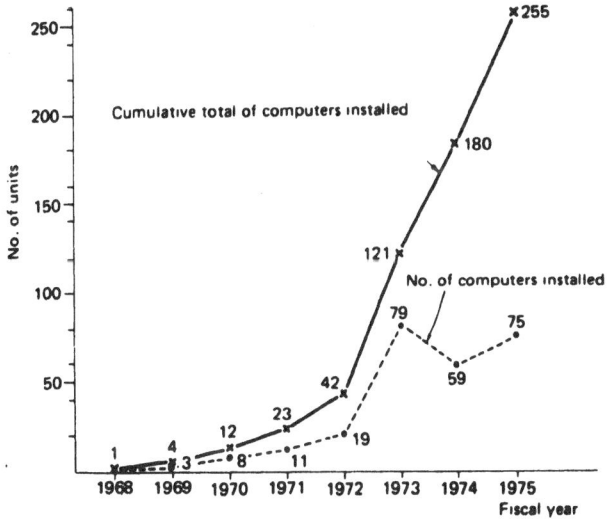

Fig. 1: Number of computers installed in Japanese hospitals.
(year of installation unknown for 13 units)

This survey was performed by the Japan Hospital Association in 1975.
The dotted line shows the annual increase in the number of hospitals
with computers and the solid line shows the accumulated number.
On the whole, the tendency of an exponential increase is noticed.

The number of hospitals having computers reached 268 in 1975, equivalent to about 10 percent of all Japanese hospitals. Figure 2 shows the size of hospitals which have computers.

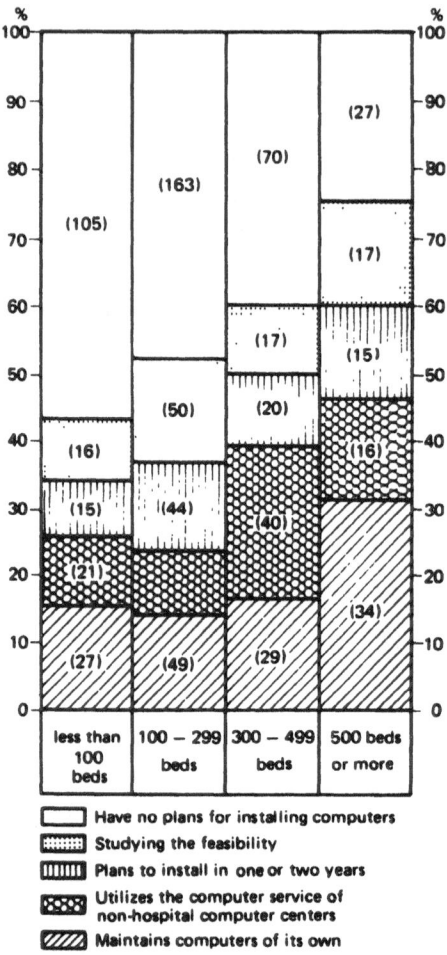

Fig. 2: State of use of computers by size of hospitals.
(Figures in parentheses indicate the number of hospitals)

This figure only shows the results from hospitals which responded to the survey; so the percentage is higher. It is seen that computers are used, regardless of the size of the hospital.

Figure 3 shows the fields of application of computers in these hospitals.

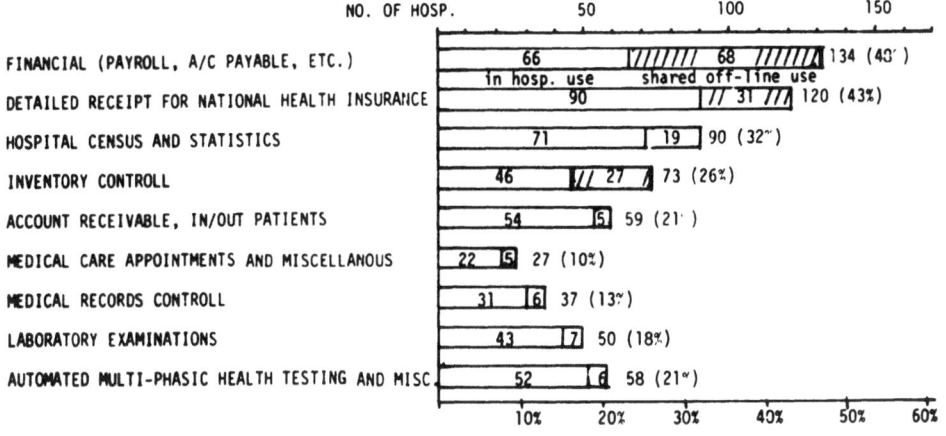

Fig. 3: Fields of application of computers in hospitals

Most of the applications are business activities applications.

Minicomputer systems are generally used for physicians' offices and big systems for large hospitals. The most sophisticated hospital information system developed àt this stage was probably the system for Komagome Hospital in Tokyo. In this hospital, about 170 terminals are placed in the wards and outpatient clinic and the doctors enter their data themselves using light pens. Almost 100% of the doctors use the terminals. Considering the fact that they are not forced to use the terminals, this figure is extremely satisfactory, even compared to the figure of the El Camino Hospital. However, this system was only developed for this particular hospital and so far has not been transferred to any other hospitals.

The government participation stage began in 1972. At that time, the concept that medical care should be regarded as a social system and the results of system sciences should be applied to seek solutions to the problems involved had gained ground. With the help of the systems approach, the optimum relationship between various medical facilities, such as clinics, hospitals and health centers, might be found. The same might be true within hospitals where the interrelationship of the various sections needs reorganization.

Acting on this hope, the Japanese Government appointed a survey team
in 1972 which investigated the application of the systems approach
to analyzing and planning health care delivery in Japan. In 1973, as
a result of this survey, a new section in the Medical Affairs
Bureau of the Ministry of Health and Welfare was established, called
the "Office for Investigating the Development of Medical Systems"
(Fig. 4).

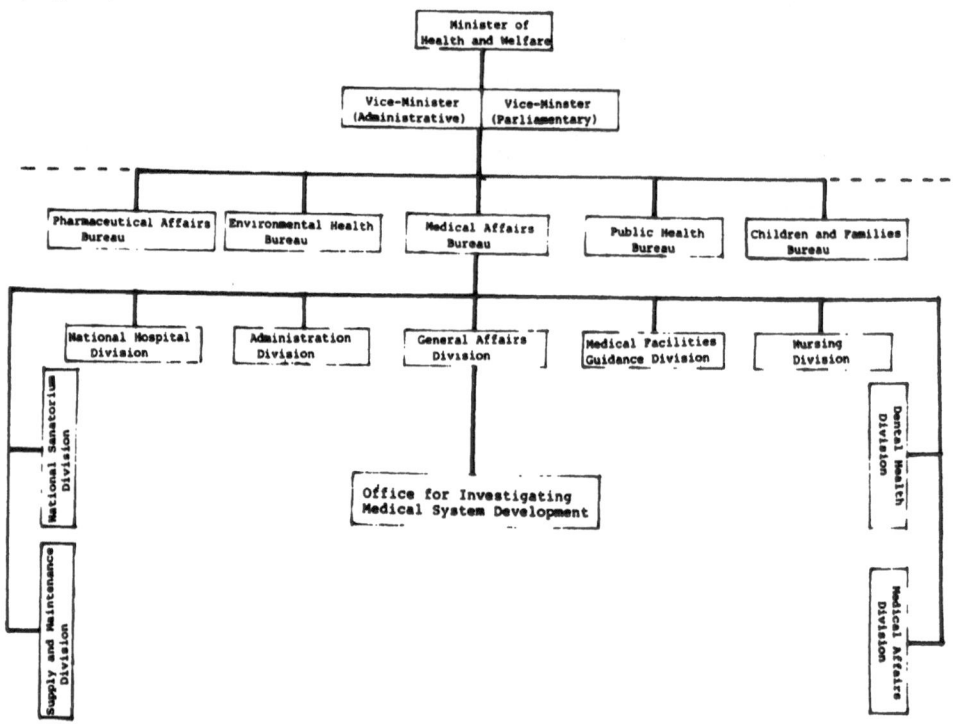

Fig. 4: Organization of the Japanese Ministry of Health and Welfare

In 1974, as a subsidiary to this office and the Ministry of
International Trade and Industry, a new organization was formed which
deals solely with the development of medical systems. Its name is the
Japanese Medical Information Systems Development Center (MEDIS-DC).

Since its establishment, the organization has supported a number of
projects. Although the budget amount was small, this fund acted as a
catalyst for the development of medical information systems. Some
representative projects are the development of the shared hospital

information systems, the development of an emergency medical
information system and the development of the data transmission
system for remote areas (Fig. 5).

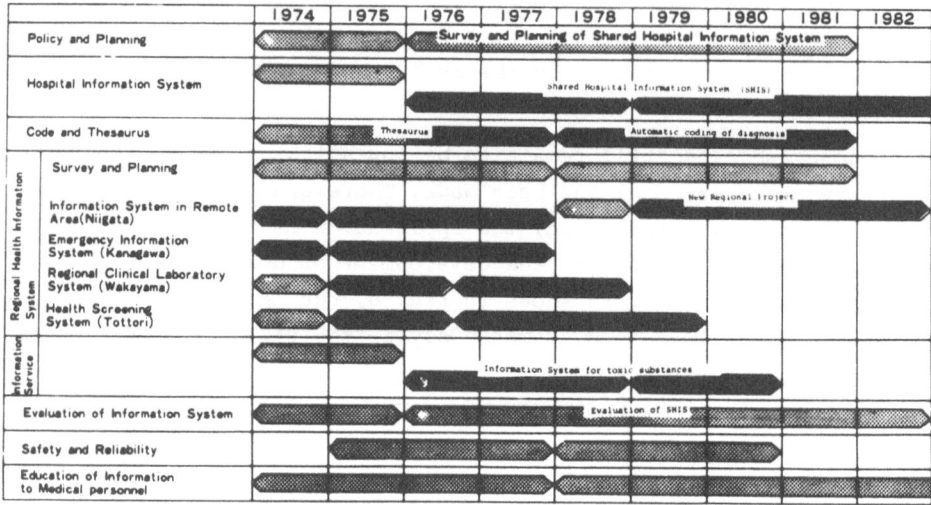

Fig. 5: Development of medical information systems by MEDIS-DC

One of the characteristics of these projects is the development of
interhospital or regional systems which could not be developed by
a single hospital.

In the Mirura Peninsula area (population 500,000), located 50 km
south of Tokyo, the emergency medical information system was
implemented. Computer terminals are placed in hospitals, clinics,
offices of medical associations and fire department (ambulance)
headquarters. Information concerning medical facilities is always
kept in the computer center. Once an emergency case is reported,
the information center searches for the most appropriate facility
and reports the name back.

In Nagasaki prefecture, located in the western part of Japan with
many isolated islands, the transmission of ECG and other medical
data over normal telephone lines is now daily routine to support
physicians working in a remote area. The shared hospital information
system is now being installed in a number of national hospitals.
It is expected that this system may promote the standardization of
medical data processing.

Although considerable progress has been achieved in technologies at the second stage, more and more attention is recently being directed to whether these systems really contribute to health care in Japan. Standardization, safety and cost-effective health care and domestic culture-oriented technologies have been important issues in recent years. This is the reason why the author believes Japan is now in the third development stage.

The above subjects still remain to be investigated and no concrete achievement or proposal has been made. Therefore, mention is made of two projects now being tried, the application of a simulation model to health care planning and the development of domestic culture-oriented technologies. As shown in Fig. 6, the national medical expenditure has increased tremendously in the past 20 years.

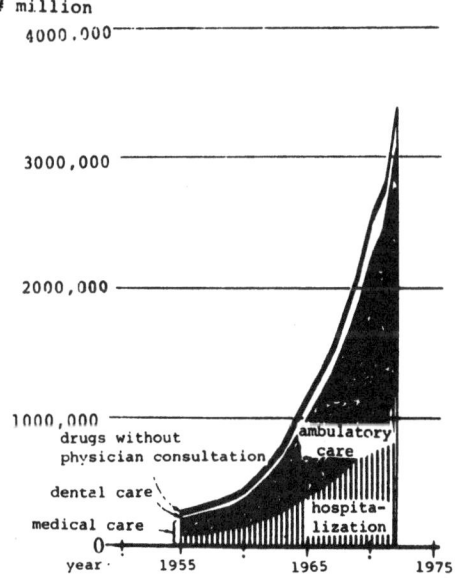

Fig. 6: National medical expenditure in the past 20 years

This increase seems to be related to both the increase in the cost per patient and the increase in the number of patients. It is still not known how to control the increase but, as a first step, it was thought worthwhile to analyze the factors related to the increase. The health care simulation model was one approach to this goal. A team was formed which was headed by the author. Because of limited space, only a summary of the results will be presented [1,2].

153

The aim of the model was to analyze the factors related to medical
demands and also, by using these factors, to predict future trends
of medical demands. Six factors were extracted: population structure,
morbidity rate, recovery rate, death rate, patient registration rate
and awareness rate. These six factors were incorporated in a
simulation model and calculation was made on how much these factors
have contributed to the increase in medical demands.
Figure 7 shows the results.

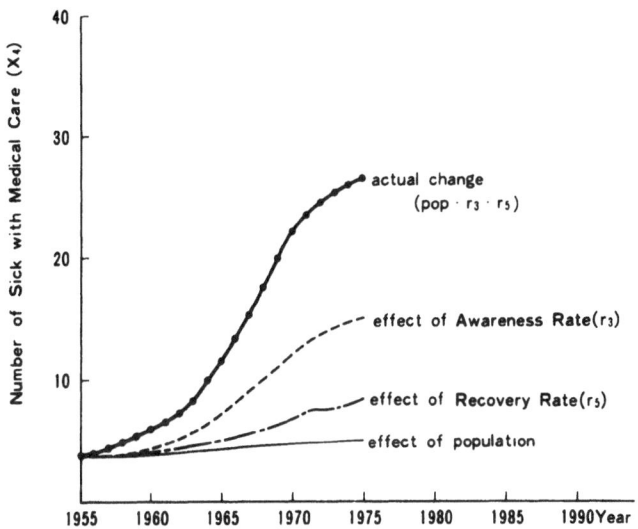

Fig. 7: Annual change of number of patients.
Effect of various factors

In the past 15 years, the awareness rate, that is the rate at which
latent patients become aware of their illnesses, increased
tremendously and contributed to the increase in the number of
patients.

This result was used for the estimation of future trends in medical demands (Fig. 8).

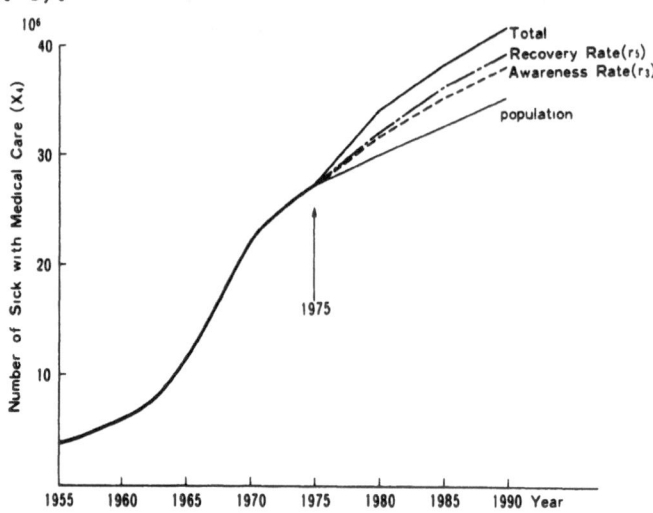

Fig. 8: Annual number of patients, estimated until 1990

Contrary to the past years, the main factor responsible for the future increase will be the change in population structure, namely, a rapid aging of the population. This is just one example of the prognoses which can be obtained from the model. These results will be helpful in planning health care on a national level.

The second important subject in this third stage is technology based on domestic culture. Japan's culture is based on Chinese ideographs for written communications, not the western alphabet. This fact has been the biggest problem when computers are used by ordinary employees. Let me briefly describe the characters or symbols used in Japan. Three types of alphabets are called katakana, hirakana and kanji. Katakana and hirakana are phonetic alphabets, made-up of 48 different symbols. Kanji are Chinese ideographs of which approximately 3,000 are used in everyday communication. Japanese written sentences are a mixture of kanji and hirakana. Katakana are only used when foreign words are cited. From the computer's standpoint, however, a Japanese line-printer can only print katakana, which are never used in ordinary sentences. This fact causes some strange difficultis. For instance, hospitals have to enter the patient's name in the insurance claim form. Since the computer can only print katakana, the claim forms printed by computers are naturally printed in katakana. However, insurance companies did not accept <u>katakana</u>-printed forms until one year ago, because the companies insisted that the names printed in <u>katakana</u> cannot correctly identify a person. Therefore, hospital personnel had to write <u>kanji</u> by hand on the computer-printed <u>katakana</u>.

This is just an example, but it will help the reader to understand that the development of computer technologies adapted to Japanese culture is very important. The Medical Information System Development Center as well as the Ministry of International Trade and Industry have been supporting the development of such technologies. At the moment, there are several devices which can print <u>kanji</u> letters. They are still too complicated to use and too expensive for a single hospital to buy. However, in such a system as the shared hospital information system, this device is implemented. It is hoped that these domestic culture-oriented technologies will be further developed in this third stage of medical computer application which has just started in Japan.

This paper described the use of computers in health care in Japan, classifying it into three stages. When looking back on the history of medical computer application in Japan, we can see that it has not been easy and progress has not been as fast as had previously been thought possible. However, based on experience, it is now surer than ever before that computer technologies will in the future contribute more and more to the improvement of health care in Japan.

<u>References</u>:

1. Kaihara, S., Fujimasa, I., Atsumi, K., Klementiev, A.:
   An approach to building a universal health care model: Morbidity
   model of degenerative diseases.
   RM-77-06, International Institute for Applied Systems Analysis,
   Laxenburg, Austria 1976.

2. Kaihara, S., Kawamura, N., Atsumi, K., Fujimasa, I.:
   Analysis and future estimation of medical demands using a health
   care model: A case study of Japan.
   RM-78-03, International Institute for Applied Systems Analysis,
   Laxenburg, Austria 1978.

Cancer Information Centers and Systems

G. Wagner

Introduction

In a field of science, which is so much in motion as is the case with
oncology, well functioning information systems are of decisive
importance. The information systems required in this domain vary
from clinical information systems of the individual hospital up to
international systems for the communication of information. The
latter, too, will have to be mentioned in this lecture, since they
represent indispensable sources of information also for cancer
control on a regional basis.

With regard to data processing, cancer research and cancer control
are in many respects still in the forefield of exact scientific
work. Data and information on cancer patients are frequently
lacking unambiguity and comparability. However, an essential
condition for gaining new knowledge in the fight against cancer is
the exchange of exactly comparable information, data and findings
on patients suffering from different forms of cancer. This demands
a standardized nomenclature of malignant tumours understood everywhere in the same way, a uniform classification of the various
forms of tumours considering the histological picture and the tumour
site, and an exact description of the tumour stage at the beginning
of treatment (if possible, supplemented by a postsurgical evaluation).
International organizations, such as CIOMS, WHO, UICC and IARC,
recognized that these are problems which can only be solved within
an international framework and have successfully devoted themselves
to these urgent tasks. In this context, I want to mention briefly
the international nomenclature project of the CIOMS aiming at a
standardization of medical terminology (4). An international working
group processes the diagnostic terms of the ICD chapter by chapter
and publishes the results in the form of individual brochures.
Roughly 400 experts from all fields of medicine, mostly university
teachers from the Federal Republic of Germany, Austria and Switzer-
land, are collaborating on the German part of the project. The

nomenclature of tumours is, of course, only a small but very important part of the entire project whose final objective is a standardized nomenclature of diagnoses with exact definitions of terms in six languages.

Some years ago, an extension of the ICD was worked out by a body of WHO experts under the leadership of the International Agency for Research on Cancer (IARC) in Lyon, namely the ICD-O (International Classification of Diseases for Oncology) (20). It represents a revision of the MOTNAC Morphology Code, a statement concerning the degree of malignancy of the respective tumour being added in a fifth digit. The German translation of this coding system, which is of great importance for a uniform tumour classification, recently appeared in book form as a "Tumor-Histologie-Schlüssel" (ICD-O-DA) (11). The German Speaking TNM Committee worked out an illustrated and extended localization code for the topography code of MOTNAC (6).[*]

Finally, the TNM system of the UICC should be mentioned in this connection (15). It attempts to exactly cover the stage and degree of spread of the different organ tumours. For this system, too, the work has not yet been completed, although translations into numerous languages are already available of those parts which have been finished.

Every national or regional cancer center will have to use the above mentioned classification systems in order to be able to submit comparable data in the future for national and international projects of cancer research and cancer control.

---

[*] Recently a revised edition, based on the ICD-O topography code, has been published. (G. Wagner (Edit.): Tumor-Lokalisations-schlüssel, 2. Auflage; Springer-Verlag, Berlin-Heidelberg, New York 1979).

National and International Cancer Information Systems

On account of the unsurveyable complexity of the biological processes
in the development of malignant tumours, modern cancer research and
cancer control with a claim to optimal efficiency can only be
carried through by national collaboration and in exchange of
experiences on an international level. However, successful cooperation is possible only if there exists a uniform stage of
development of the participating institutions. A well functioning
net of information systems, which is able to communicate the latest
state of the art fast and selectively to all physicians and
scientists concerned with the cancer problem, is of decisive
importance in this connection.

Realizing this problem, the USA - within the framework of their
National Cancer Program (13) - attributed great importance to the
development of cancer information systems and centers and provided
considerable funds for this purpose. The National Cancer Act of 1971
contains directives which gave new impulses to the formulation and
formalization of information services in the cancer field. For
example, Section 407 reads as follows:

> The Act authorizes the Director, NCI, to:
> "Collect, analyze, and disseminate all data useful in the
> prevention, diagnosis, and treatment of cancer, including
> the establishment of an international cancer research
> data bank to collect, catalog, store, and disseminate
> insofar as feasible the results of cancer research
> undertaken in any country for the use of any person
> involved in cancer research in any country".

> In Section 410, it further authorizes the Director, NCI, to:
> "Take necessary action to ensure that all channels for the
> dissemination and exchange of scientific knowledge and
> information are maintained between the National Cancer
> Institute and other scientific, medical, and biomedical
> disciplines and organizations nationally and internationally".

The International Cancer Research Data Bank (ICRDB) Program (14)
developed during the last few years, which serves the exchange of
experiences and the dissemination of information on an international
level and obtains information from numerous sources, is made up
of a large number of subsystems which contribute information on

cancer with varying aims and in different fields of oncology. The "Current Cancer Research Project Analysis Center" (CCRESPAC) was the first of five projected "Cancer Information Dissemination and Analysis Centers" to be established within the framework of this program. It collects, catalogues and evaluates information on on-going cancer research projects. The Smithsonian Science Exchange (SSIE) has been designated to operate this service. Scientists reporting on-going projects to CCRESPAC will, in turn, be served with reference journals published within the framework of ICRDB, e.g. the Special Listings on Current Cancer Research, which pick out a certain subject of cancer research each month, or the Cancergrams which appear monthly and contain papers on certain topics selected from more than 1,500 journals.

A specialized project within the framework of ICRDB, established jointly by the International Agency for Research on Cancer (IARC) in Lyon and the German Cancer Research Center (DKFZ) in Heidelberg and funded at a rate of 50% from means of the ICRDB program, is the "Clearing-House for On-going Research in Cancer Epidemiology". The Clearing-House collects information on on-going, i.e. not yet completed,research projects in the field of cancer epidemiology on a worldwide basis and makes this information available to interested scientists in the form of annual "Directories". It is the aim of this project to communicate pertinent information in the broad field of cancer epidemiology, to establish personal contacts between researchers working on the same sector and to help to avoid,wherever possible, duplication and multiplication of research activities. The first volume which appeared in 1976 contained information on 622 projects from 65 countries; the annual volume for 1977 contained 905 projects from 70 countries; the volume for 1978 covered 1,092 projects from 67 countries (12). Several tables of contents, among them two permuted indexes, will facilitate the use of the Directory. There are close connections and a regular exchange of information between the Clearing-House and CCRESPAC as well as the UICC Clearing-House for Controlled Clinical Trials in Paris.

CANCERLINE is a further information system which should be mentioned within the framework of ICRDB. CANCERLINE is a computer-based information system for search and retrieval of abstracts related to cancer research. It consists of three data bases:

- CANCERLIT;
- CANCERPROJ and
- CLINPROT.

CANCERLIT (CANCER LITerature) contains 80,000 abstracts of published cancer literature dealing with all aspects of cancer reseach. It is updated monthly and will grow at a rate of approximately 25,000 abstracts per year.

CANCERPROJ (CANCER PROJects) contains 16,000 descriptions of on-going cancer research projects collected from cancer researchers worldwide.

CLINPROT (CLINical PROTocols) contains nearly 1,000 summaries of clinical protocols for treating specific types of cancer including specific anticancer agents or modalities. It is updated every three months.

A system comparable to CANCERLIT, but considerably older and more extensive than the latter, is the cancer literature information system CANCERNET (formerly SABIR-C) which has been developed jointly by the French Cancer Research Center in Villejuif and the German Cancer Research Center in Heidelberg (18). Within the framework of this system more than 1,200 medical journals are evaluated; the papers on cancer contained therein are indexed according to given rules and the key-words characterizing the contents of the papers together with the usual bibliographic data are covered and stored. At a yearly input of between 12,000 and 15,000 papers, the CANCERNET databank presently contains more than 100,000 titles which are available for searches of any kind. The CANCERNET thesaurus contains more than 5,000 preferred terms and roughly 12,000 minor terms which may be purposefully searched for in German, English and French. In Heidelberg the entire data base is stored index-sequentially on disks with a record length of at most 1,500 characters. Additionally, there is an inverted file in which the document number of each article dealing with the key-word in question is assigned to the latter. The search for any desired number of key-words or key-word combinations in the data base as it presently stands takes but a few seconds.

The relevant titles of a search may be printed either in the form of lists or index cards.

In 1977, about 1,500 searches were dealt with in our institute for physicians and scientists from the Federal Republic of Germany, the German Democratic Republic and Austria; besides, there were more than 450 permanent orders in the field of "selective dissemination of information". About one third of the search inquiries concerned basic research in the field of oncology (for example, chemical carcinogenesis, biochemistry, viral research, experimental cytology); about two thirds pertained to the field of clinical oncology (in particular the tumours of the breast and the female genital organs, the gastro-intestinal tract and the respiratory organs). Roughly half of the inquiries originated from universities, about a quarter from extra-universitary research institutions; the remainder is divided between practitioners and hospital physicians, authorities, associations and the pharmaceutical industry.

In the meantime, the countries Italy, Yugoslavia and Poland affiliated to the original axis Paris-Heidelberg *). In this way, a cancer literature information network has come about which befits the new name CANCERNET. The concept of CANCERNET provides that the countries concerned contribute their relevant literature to the system; in turn, they receive, by way of monthly exchange, the entire material stored in the system. CANCERNET represents the prototype of a well functioning international cooperation in the field of electronic information retrieval on the medical sector (18).

At present an extensive international cancer research program with an information base for the countries of the COMECON block, comparable to the ICRDB program, is under development in the USSR (3).

---

*) In 1979 Japan joined the system.

Regional Cancer Information Centers

Improving the quality of life is one of the most essential problems
of today's health care. In 1975, the 28th World Health Assembly
gave out this password as its program of action and set priorities
for its future work. These include, apart from the continuing
eradication of infectious diseases, the elimination of hunger and
malnutrition and the improved care for mother and child,
environmental sanitation, primarily involving air pollution, water
supply and sewage disposal. In the field of environmental pollution,
cancer is today considered to be the most important identified
hazard (10). All civilized nations took legislative steps during
the last few years in order to protect our endangered environment,
for instance, in the USA, the Clean Air Act, the Federal Water
Pollution Control Act, the Safe Drinking Water Act, the Toxic
Substances Control Act, the Federal Insecticide, Fungicide and
Rodenticide Act and the Pure Food and Drug Act. The Delaney Clause
of the latter that set a zero tolerance limit for carcinogenic food
additives has lately become a focal point of criticism, e.g., in
connection with the Saccharin affair.

Among the carcinogenic factors identified up to this day, those of
our environment are by far the most important ones. However, this
does not merely concern the substances in our "macro-environment" -
i.e. air, water, food, and other pollutants - but also our "micro-
environment" - our personal life style including our eating,
drinking, and smoking habits. While our governments are responsible
for keeping our macro-environment clean, we ourselves are called
upon to avoid carcinogenic substances in our micro-environment.

The fight against cancer today does not dissipate itself merely in
basic research and the development of new diagnostic and
therapeutic methods. In addition, it requires a health policy and
organizational measures, provision of funds for prevention and
early detection, the development of new strategies for in-patient
and out-patient care and aftercare for cancer patients in modern
regional systems (1), medical training as well as health education
of the population.

It cannot be expected that, in the foreseeable future, there will
be fundamentally new methods of treatment in the field of cancer
or that existing methods will be considerably improved. An
improvement in the results of treatment can, therefore, only be

achieved by the integration of the knowledge of oncological experts
from various disciplines and by an intensivation of early
detection and early treatment. We know today that the first
treatment of a cancer patient frequently is his only chance of
being cured. It is, therefore, the aim of our endeavours to give
each patient in whom a cancer has been diagnosed the optimal
therapy according to the present state of the art as early as
possible. The present structure of our health care services does not
warrant fulfilment of this demand. It is obvious that better
results can be achieved in treatment centers specially set up for
cancer patients than in institutions which do not specialize in
this field. For more than ten years a change in the system of
cancer therapy has, therefore, been discussed in numerous countries
and has partly been put into practice. Thus, for example, it was
decided in France in 1970 to set up regional centers for cancer
control, cancer treatment, and cancer research (5). In Great
Britain, too, a Committee of the Central Health Service Council
proposed in 1970 to set up a network of regional oncological centers
within certain large hospitals (2). In Norway, four special cancer
therapy centers were established in different parts of the country
by a governmental order in 1970; similar activities are underway
in Denmark and Sweden (7, 8). In 1973 a Working Group of the WHO
Europe concerned itself with the subject "The Organization of
Comprehensive Cancer Control Programmes" (19). In numerous other
countries (including the Federal Republic of Germany) such tumour
centers are now about to be built up (9).

In the USA, the analogous concept of the so-called "Comprehensive
Cancer Centers" has been developed. The M.D. Anderson Hospital
and Tumor Institute in Houston, the Roswell Park Memorial Institute
in Buffalo, and the Memorial Sloan-Kettering Institute in New York
served as models for such CCC's. In 1968 there already existed 15
such centers. Within the framework of the National Cancer Act,
their number is to be increased to 33 by 1980; each of these
centers is then to provide for one certain region.

In the interest of facilitating the development and setting up
of specialized cancer treatment centers, the Committee on
International Collaborative Activities (CICA) of the International
Union against Cancer (UICC) issued a "Handbook for Developing a
Comprehensive Cancer Centre" in September 1977 which takes its
bearings substantially from US-American experiences (17).

Under the paragraph "General Operating Concept" we find:

"Comprehensive cancer centres do not work in isolation,
but rather extend their activities to influence the
community and region. The good-will and confidence of
the community, of area physicians, and of patients are
essential to a centre's success. The centre must earn
a reputation for expertise - the generation and coordination
of new information".

One of the tasks of such regional cancer treatment centers, apart
from safeguarding the optimal therapy for the individual patient
according to present knowledge as well as guaranteeing a controlled
follow-up and, where necessary, rehabilitation of the patient, is
therapeutic research (e.g., the development of new chemo-
therapeutical treatment schemes, gaining new epidemiological
knowledge, the coordination and provision of the most recent results
of research, etc.). All these tasks can only be fulfilled with the
aid of an efficient information center, equipped with the instruments
of modern data processing. Figure 1 shows the central function and

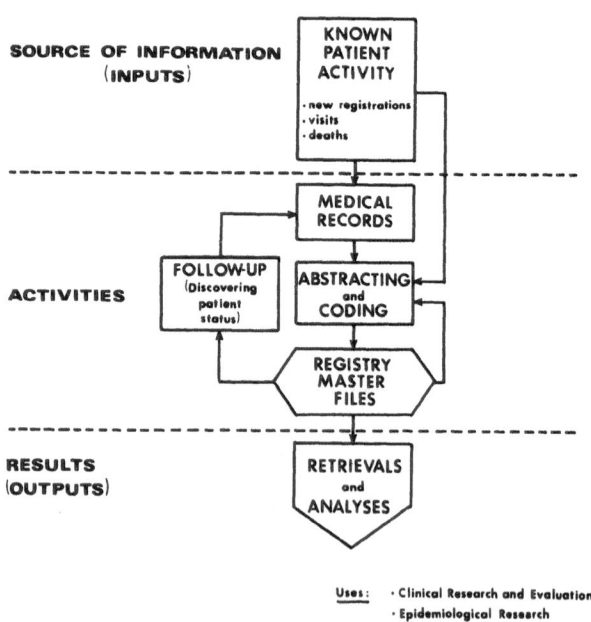

Fig. 1: The functions on the Information center within a Cancer
Treatment Center (from (17)).

importance of such an information center - frequently called "Clinical Cancer Registry" - within the framework of a cancer treatment center.

It is the task of clinical documentation to cover the clinical picture of the individual patient as exactly as possible, to record any findings secured during the patient's stay in the hospital and to follow up the further fate of the patient as completely as possible. An essential prerequisite for this is a documentation system set up in the form of special data bases or data banks, accessible to authorized persons only and thus guaranteeing sufficient data protection, which has to allow a continuous care and observation of patients for at least 10 years following treatment. It must be warranted that the physicians of the tumour center concerned and the practitioners involved in the follow-up of the patient will have constant access to their patients' data.

Furthermore, such an information center should provide useful data for comparative investigations (within and between the tumour centers of a country, but also internationally) and should also allow for a "medical audit".

A uniform data acquisition suitable for EDP should, in our opinion, consist of a generally accepted basic program (minimum basic oncological data set), to which, according to the type of tumour, further information (special oncological documentation) will have to be added. The standardized basic documentation will have to be worked out by a committee on which all model centers are represented and should be declared obligatory for all tumor centers so that comparability of the most important basic data of the various centers and a common analysis of these data is possible at any time.

The clinical documentation must be set up in such a manner as to allow additional information from other sources to be unmistakably assigned to it via an identification item permitting an exact record linkage.

It is a further important task of the tumour centers to set up standardized therapy programs. The type of treatment of a cancer patient must no longer depend upon the sort of hospital to which he has been primarily admitted - more or less by chance. The same therapy, adapted to the latest state of the art, should be available to patients everywhere. A constant collaboration of

clinical experts will be required in order to keep therapy programs
updated. Provisions will have to be made to ensure suitable
dissemination of the knowledge about these programs.

Finally, the information center should be responsible for the
organization of patient follow-up, for keeping the appointments for
re-examinations and for updating patient-oriented information. It
should safeguard the contact between out-patient department and
practitioner and analyze the data and information collected, as
required. For example, it will be an important task to establish
average survival times or five-year survival rates for the various
organ tumours dependent on sex and age of the patient, on the stage
of the disease, on the type of tumour, kind of therapy etc.

A scheme of the information flow in such an information center is
shown in Figure 2.

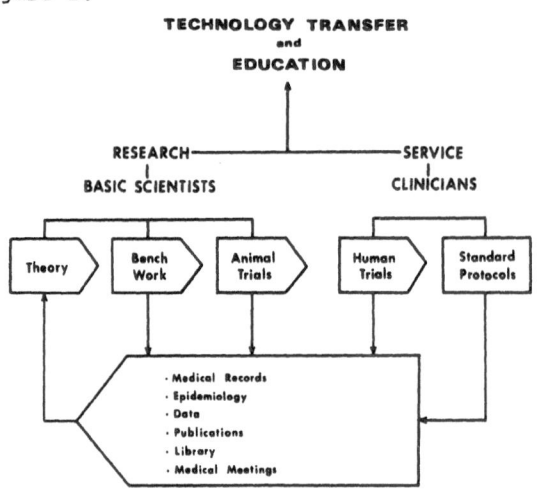

Fig. 2: Flow of Information within the Cancer Treatment
        Center (from (17)).

A further important feature of the cancer treatment centers is their
"community outreach responsibility", i.e. the coordination of
therapy programs in regional collaboration with other hospitals,
the appointment of specialists as consultants for smaller
hospitals and, last not least, the inclusion of the general
practitioner in a regional patient care system. As a primary filter
for cancer patients in the population, the general practitioner
plays an important part, also in the model of the oncological
center. Thus, an optimal follow-up is only possible through
collaboration between the cancer center and the general practitioner.

Therefore, every cancer treatment center must strive to gain a regionally attractive position as a center of information and training for general practitioners.

The tumour centers which are now being developed everywhere will only function optimally if they build up their data acquisition and evaluation systems according to internationally agreed, comparable criteria and will thus be able to measure their own successes and failures by international standards.

In order to gain experiences about the international exchange of data on cancer patients, the UICC developed an "International Cancer Patient Data Exchange System" (ICPDS) in which a total of twelve large cancer centers in the USA, in Western and Eastern Europe are taking part. The program provides for the acquisition of certain patient data for five organ cancers to start with (breast, colon, rectum, larynx carcinoma and Hodgkin's disease).

Changes in findings or results of therapy will be reported at six-monthly intervals (16). Computer centers were established in Houston and Brussels for the exchange of data on an international level. A similar project has meanwhile been developed for the Comprehensive Cancer Centers in the USA (21).

I have attempted to show the present state of development of cancer information centers and systems. In so doing, I am aware of the fact that this survey is incomplete and, in view of the speed of development, cannot possibly be "comprehensive". However, I do hope that I succeeded in demonstrating how numerous and varied the efforts are which are made on this sector and which importance is attributed to the cancer problem worldwide.

References

1. Albert, R.E., Train, R.E., Anderson, E.: Rationale Developed by the Environment Protection Agency for the Assessment of Carcinogenic Risks. J.nat.Cancer Inst. 58 (1977) 1537-1541.

2. Central Health Services Council: On Cancer Organization. In: Annual Report for the Year 1970. London: H.M. Stat.Office 1971.

3. Cerkovnyi, G.F.: The Soviet System of Statistical Information on Cancer. Meeting on Cancer Statistics Information Subsystems, Minsk, USSR, 6.-10. Sept. 1976.

4. CIOMS: Provisional International Nomenclature, Vols 1-5. Geneva: CIOMS 1972 ff.

5. Denoix, P.: Originalité des centres anti-cancéreux francais. Typescript, Institut Gustave-Roussy, 1966.

6. Deutschsprachiger TNM-Ausschuß: Tumor-Lokalisationsschlüssel des Deutschsprachigen TNM-Ausschuß. Heidelberg: Deutsches Krebsforschungszentrum 1974.

7. Einhorn, J., Larsson, L.G.: Cancersjukvaardens och radioterapins organisation. Läkartidn. 67 (1970) 1181 ff.

8. Eker, R.: Det Norske Radium Hospital. En analyse av funksjoner og behov. Plan for utvidelse og ombygging. Oslo 1968.

9. German Cancer Research Center: Memorandum on the Establishment of a Comprehensive Cancer Center (CCC) in Heidelberg. Typescript, Heidelberg 1976.

10. Higginson, J.: A Hazardous Society? Individual versus Community Responsibility in Cancer Prevention. Amer.J.publ.Hlth 66 (1976) 359-366.

11. Jacob, W., Scheida, D., Wingert, F. (Hrsg.): Tumor-Histologie-Schlüssel - ICD-O-DA. Berlin-Heidelberg-New York: Springer 1978.

12. Muir, S., Wagner, G. (Eds): Directory of On-going Research in Cancer Epidemiology 1977. IARC Scientific Publ. No. 17. Lyon: Internat.Agency for Research on Cancer 1977.

13. National Cancer Institute: National Cancer Program - Cancer Information Services. - Concept Paper, March, 1973, Typescript.

14. National Cancer Institute: Plans for the International Cancer Research Data Bank (ICRDB) Program of the National Cancer Institute, USA. June 14, 1974. Typescript.

15. UICC: TNM Classification of Malignant Tumours. Second Edition.
Geneva: UICC 1974.

16. UICC: Ad hoc CICA Working Party to plan the Development of
International Cancer Patient Data Exchange Systems (ICPDS).
Typescript 1977.

17. UICC - Committee on International Activities: Handbook for
Developing a Comprehensive Cancer Centre.
Typescript, Sept. 1977.

18. Wagner, G., Sandor, L.: Das Krebsliteratur-Informationssystems
CANCERNET. Med.uns.Zeit 2 (1978) 40-47.

19. WHO: The Organization of Comprehensive Cancer Control Programs -
Report of a Working Group, Oslo, 22.-24. Nov. 1972.
Document WHO Euro 8102/1973.

20. WHO: ICD-O. International Classification of Diseases for
Oncology, 1976. Geneva, World Health Organization 1976.

21. _____: Centralized Cancer Patient Data System - Data Acquisition
Manual (August 1977). Typescript.

Technology for the Health of a Nation: Radiant Imaging

G.S. Lodwick

The newer radiant imaging technologies, principally those which are
displayed in digital format such as computerized tomography, nuclear
scanning, ultrasonic scanning, and the new permutations of computerized tomography, emission tomography and ultrasound tomography, have
become a highly significant element of the health care of our nation.
The major impact of these technologies has been in improved diagnosis
and patient management. The cost of these digital technologies in
1977 was estimated to be slightly more than two billion dollars, and
is now predicted to be two and a half billion dollars by the end of
1980 (1). The need for controlling the cost of health care has figured
prominently in public policy debates on national health insurance.
If national health insurance were to be adopted in the United States
it is believed that the demand for these and other new techniques
will raise costs to even higher levels. The sum of health care costs
for the United States in 1978 were in the domain of $ 180 billion
dollars, placing the total cost of imaging at only 1.1% of the total.
This is a rather small proportion of the cost, considering the values
returned (4).

Computerized tomography has been a major focus of attention in
efficacy studies pertaining to reducing the cost of health care. The
latest generation of CT scanners, some of which now provide excellent
digital arrays of 512 x 512 pixels and scanning times of from one to
two seconds, have installation costs of nearly one million dollars per
unit. Early estimates were that there would be more than two thousand
CT scanners in operation in the United States by 1980. The facts are
that only 1,000 were installed by 1978, and that new orders have
dropped off precipitously. This trend has largely been due to the
fact that CT, while exciting, is initially very expensive, and was
marketed before its efficacy in the diagnostic process was known.
Forecasting sales trends in the diagnostic imaging systems market,
according to a CSI study (2), indicate that the sales in the scanner
sector of the market would peak by 1978 and decline until at least

1983. Although growth in non-U.S. markets would partially offset
these losses, scanner sales have been predicted to flatten by 1982.
Government legislation and review committee regulations have played
a significant role in arresting the development of the diagnostic
imaging systems market. In the year between July 1976 and July 1977,
State review agencies rejected 35% of the proposed purchases of CT
scanners, and the record indicates that the trend is continuing.

According to the Arthur D. Little report concerning computing
tomography versus alternative diagnostic procedures (Table 1), CT
scanning could be shown to displace a substantial proportion of
other complimentary imaging procedures, particularly pneumoencephalography and nuclear scans of the brain. As the result of this and
other studies, it has also been predicted that computerized tomography
of the head, through improved diagnosis could reduce the costs of
exploratory surgery by $ 500 million dollars in the 1980's. However,

Table 1: Use of Alternative Diagnostic Procedures, Total Cost
Cranial, Abdominal and Mediastinal Diagnoses.
(Reprinted from Arthur D.Little, Inc., Comparative Cost
Analysis: Computed Tomography versus Alternative Diagnostic
Procedures 1977 and 1980).

Diagnostic Modality	CT Not Available	CT Available	
	1977	1977	1980
	(millions)	(millions)	(millions)
Computed Tomography	----	$ 381.9	$ 1,018.5
Conventional X-ray *)	$ 503.0	503.0	461.9
Special X-ray Procedures *)	713.0	632.5	568.3
Nuclear Medicine	676.5	524.0	457.6
Ultrasound	120.6	120.6	108.6
Exploratory Surgery	1,033.4	992.9	516.6
	$ 3,046	$ 3,171	$ 3,132

*) Pneumoencephalography and angiography

as has been pointed out by Evens (4), the realization of these cost
savings may not be possible because an insufficient number of
computerized tomographic units will be available in time to provide
such cost savings. As of today, the proportional costs of CT imaging
in the United States is less than .3% of the total bill for health
care. The evidence has indicated that body tomography may have a
very significant impact in diagnosis, particularly of obscure
abdominal problems. Through its ability to provide direct measurements of radiation absorption by tissue, CT becomes a major element
of a combined computed tomography/radiation therapy treatment planning
system. The basic research and development for such a program has
been carried out at the University of Missouri (3) and is now being
marketed by a major manufacturer. The importance of computerized
tomography would now seem to be somewhat underestimated by the
health care providers who are concerned primarily in initial costs.

Ultrasound

Ultrasound scanning is now the most rapidly developing imaging
discipline. Many new ultrasound scanners are being equipped with
digital scan converters which generate digital arrays of 512 x 512
pixel size, each point of the array representing from six to eight
bits of information. It is estimated that from twenty to thirty
patients per day can be scanned with an estimated 15 scans per
patient. Images can be stored on a digital device such as magnetic
tape or discs, although the current mode of physician viewing is
through the use of Polaroid or film images with multiple images on
each film. Ultrasound scanners now range in price of between
$ 40,000 to $ 90,000 for real time sector scanners, while more
technologically sophisticated phased array scanners range to well
over $ 100,000 in cost. The increasing demand for use of ultrasound
is divided between diagnostic radiology, obstetrics and gynecology,
and cardiology for real time cardiac and vascular scanning. Ultrasound has proved to be an inexpensive, non-invasive, and safe
modality; highly successful with certain examinations. For example,
it is the least expensive and fastest imaging examination for
determining the presence of gall stones. The previously referred
to CSI report indicates that with new developments in real time
scanning, ultrasound scanners will lead the market in sales growth
with compound yearly increases approaching 28% by 1982. It is
believed that by 1982, ultrasound imaging will constitute the most

significant sector of the new imaging market with annual sales
approaching $ 300 million dollars. As with CT scanner suppliers,
CSI predicts that vendors of ultrasound imaging equipment will
experience a major shakedown that will eliminate almost all competi-
tors excepting those with interest in other imaging technologies.

Nuclear Imaging

Nuclear imaging is recognized as a diagnostic technology which offers
a physiologic kind of clinical assessment of disease which is not
possible with many other imaging modalities. Emission tomography,
for example,while still in the prototype stage is able to demonstrate
the site of uptake of physiological tracers in the brain, providing
a kind of information about the location of cerebral activity which
never before has been accessible (11). Nuclear scanning of the
skeleton is a major and valuable source of information which
complements, and in some instances, replaces the need for routine
radiographic imaging. Nuclear physiologic studies of the cardiovascular system are rapidly growing in importance. CSI has reported
that nuclear medical products will integrate with computers to form
new products that promise to complement CT scanners.

Other Imaging Technologies

In the United States, experience with thermographic imaging in breast
cancer screening has been very disappointing, owing to the low
sensitivity and specificity of this examination for the detection
of cancer. Computer pattern recognition technology is being used
to improve the diagnostic quality of thermographic imaging (13, 14).
While results are promising, they have not yet materialized into a
clinically useful tool.

With radiographic imaging, research is being carried out in the use
of solid state detectors coupled with computer systems with the
objective of producing digital images which are generated directly
and stored electronically without being recorded on film. Another
major advance is dynamic radiographic imaging with digital image
enhancement and subtraction technology that has been developed by
Mistretta and others (5, 12) for the imaging of low density
contrast studies. Such examinations show promise of successful
imaging of the heart and coronary vessels without the use of cardiac
catheterization.

Image Storage

Image Storage is an ever-increasing problem, not just for radiographic images but also for CT, ultrasound, and nuclear medicine
images. The University of Missouri's MARS (Missouri Automated
Radiology System) radiology information system provides excellent
retrieval of radiographic-image files, but the mix of tapes, disks,
films, and other digital and analog recording media presents a
problem of greater magnitude, where the desired information may be
somewhere on a magnetic tape. Further, storage of CT images provides
only that information thought important by the first examiner.

The resolution of all such technical problems must inevitably
satisfy the requirement of quality patient care. Radiologists and
a wide variety of specialists with patient care responsibilities
need to see and compare such images to better understand their
patients'problems.

The transmission and display characteristics of the newer imaging
technologies may help resolve the storage and retrieval problem,
with the cost increase, it is hoped, offset by improved diagnostic
accuracy. The new image information can be stored on high-density
video or digital disks, or can be automatically recorded on film
or paper with a flying spot scanner (6). Images so stored could
be digitally retrieved under computer control and displayed at
viewing stations where the radiologist can combine the information
from several complementary imaging modalities. Problems to be
resolved are standardization, development of display technologies
capable of reproducing the diagnostic content of radiographs, the
production of electronic images that can effectively eliminate the
need for x-ray films as we know them, and the design and testing
of viewing facilities with sufficient flexibility and speed to be
acceptable to the radiologist user. All of these problems, including
the entire image management system, are under investigation.
However, until such a system is available and cost effective,
radiologists will continue to struggle with their own solutions
to the storage problem.

This paper provides but a glimpse of the new imaging technologies
which are having a positive impact on the quality of health care.
With the rapid technological development which is possible today,
new imaging technologies can be produced and marketed before

efficacy studies have been carried out. This on occasion, can
provide a technology which is evolving for an application. As a
result, the National Institutes of Health have sponsored efficacy
studies to show the comparative usefulness of new technologies for
the diagnosis of specific diseases in specific areas of the body.
Some such studies are expected to soon have an impact on the cost
of health care,through providing better indicators of which imaging
technology is more useful in which situation. The overall picture,
however, is one of an explosion of new radiant images which provide
for much greater insight into disease than mere morphology. This
new insight, which is in the domain of normal and abnormal physiology
and biochemistry; considered with advances in computer information
management (7, 10) and diagnosis (8, 9) has introduced a golden era
to radiology and to medicine.

References

1. Comparative Cost Analysis: Computed Tomography versus Alternative
   Diagnostic Procedures, 1977 and 1980. (Cambridge, Mass.:
   Arthur D. Little, Inc., 1977).

2. Diagnostic Imaging: CT and Ultrasound. Study done by Creative
   Strategies International, Sunnyvale, Calif. 1979.

3. Edwards, M., Keller, J., Larsen, G., Hagemeyer, D., Bull, S.,
   Carter, D., Roberg, A., Rafferty, P., Patta, S., Sandler, B.,
   Whitaker, F.: Design, operation and initial testing of a computed
   tomography-radiation therapy treatment planning system utilizing
   a whole body CT scanner, (submitted for publication).

4. Evens, Ronald, Mallinckrodt Institute of Radiology, Washington
   University School of Medicine: Personal communication.

5. Houk, T.L., Kruger, R.A., Mistretta, C.A., Riederer, S.M.,
   Shaw, C., Lancaster, J.C., Flemming, D.: Real-time digital
   K-edge subtraction fluoroscopy. Invest. Radiol. 14 (1979) 270-278.

6. Lodwick, G.S.: Professional platform: Has microfilming failed as
   a method of storage and retrieval of radiologic-image information?
   Appl. Radiol. 9 (1980) 18.

7. Lodwick, G.S.: On using a diagnostic simulator to detect causes of error, (to be presented at Third International Symposium on Planning of Radiological Departments, Amsterdam, June, 1980).

8. Lodwick, G.S., Wilson, A.J., Farrell, C., Virtama, P., Dittrich, F.: Determining growth rates of focal lesions of bone from radiographs. Radiology 134 (1980) 577-583.

9. Lodwick, G.S., Wilson, A.J., Farrell, C., Virtama, P., Smeltzer, F.M., Dittrich, F.: Estimating rate of growth in bone lesions: Observer performance and error. Radiology 134 (1980) 585-590.

10. Lodwick, G.S., Wickizer, C.R., Dickhaus, E.: Tenth anniversary of operational MARS: Its future, (submitted for publication in Meth.Inform.Med.).

11. Reivich, M., Kuhl, D., Wolf, A., Greenberg, J., Phelps, M., Ido, T., Casella, V., Fowler, J., Hoffman, E., Alavi, A., Som, P., Sokoloff, L.: The ^{18}F fluorodeoxyglucose method for the measurement of local cerebral glucose utilization in man. Circ.Res. 44 (1979) 127-137.

12. Ritman, E.L., Sturm, E., Wood, E.H.: A biplane roentgen videometry system for dynamic (60/second) studies of the shape and size of circulatory structures, particularly the left ventricle. In P.H.Heintzen (Edit.): Roentgen-, Cin- and Videodensitometry, pp. 179-211. (Stuttgart: G. Thieme 1971).

13. Rose, J.L., Good, M.S., Goldbert, B.B.: Ultrasonic pattern recognition potential for the early detection of breast cancer, (presented at Fourth International Symposium on Ultrasonic Imaging and Tissue Characterization, June, 1979).

14. Shaber, G.S.: Final Report - Evaluation of Thermography in Mass Screening for Breast Cancer. NCI-NO1-CN-35027, July, 1979.

Inpatient Health Care Delivery Models

J. Anderson and A. Nimalasuriya

Introduction

The inpatient model of the medical information system as it has been
developed either as the traditional medical record, the Weed problem-
oriented record [4] or the decision-directed record [1] or one or
other members of the family of medical records [2,3], will be
discussed. The implementation used here will reflect our work in
medical inpatient information systems related either to the decision-
directed record or to the Weed problem-oriented record. At present we
are doing comparative experiments with both types of record. The basic
model of information about hospital inpatients, despite the difference
in objectives and details of formulating the information derived from
the real situation, is the same. This presentation reviews eight basic
modules and their different segments, which deal with the medical information created and used to guide and monitor care during the
patients stay in hospital. Both logical and relational analysis and
procedures have been used in decomposing the information system and
in the design of new models.

Communication Module

This is an important first module for it reflects the way in which
the patient becomes an inpatient and includes basic data about the
patients identity. He may reach the hospital as an emergency patient
either referred by social agencies such as the police or if he has
fallen in a public place or been involved in an accident. He may also
be referred as an emergency admission by his general practitioner or
other doctor, usually with a brief but prior warning to the hospital.
There may or may not be patient identification data or information
about the disorder and any treatment given. Other patients may be
referred to hospital for an opinion about their clinical condition
and the hospital doctor then arranged for an emergency admission.
Other patients are referred for inpatient care from routine waiting
lists, usually following a visit or visits to an outpatient
department or policlinic. Basically there will be either no
communication or identification or partial or complete identification

and clinical data. The patient may or may not be able to give
information himself depending on his state of consciousness, but this
is usually obtained from an accompanying person, family or the next
of kin. Thus the initial encounter involves a variable information
transfer but it is important to have as much information as possible
to prevent errors of diagnosis and clinical management.

Admission Module

The data about patient identification, including name, home address,
data of birth and religion are obtained from the patient or his
relatives by medical, nursing or lay staff. Depending on the type of
health service and the insurance system in operation the first
contact may not be clinical but a financial assessor who decides if
the patient can be accepted as an inpatient after proving his
financial status. Usually admission data is obtained about the name
and address of his doctor and his next of kin. His marital status and
occupation or occupation of the husband, if the female patient is
married, is given. Note is made of the type of admission whether
immediate, waiting list, transferred from another hospital, etc.
Several identification system numbers may be required such as previous
hospital number or insurance or social security number or the individual's health insurance number.

This forms the basic identification data for the patient during his
stay in hospital. It is usually linked together with the record by a
hospital or other identification number. By means of this number it is
then possible to get the total basic data about a patient on
admission.

So far discussion has centred on the type of data input to the
information system. Such data is, however, used to check the patients
identification with a master list of previous inpatients and, if
necessary, to retrieve previous hospital identification numbers. This
enables past records to be obtained, if required. The master index can
also be used to link the patient to insurance system and initiate the
necessary audit trail for payment for services. The information about
religion allows the information system to tell priests and padres
about the members of their faith admitted to hospital. The doctor's
name and address is essential for the communication which may take
place either during the patients stay or on discharge from the hospital.

Thus the data needed in admission module are related to information that will be output from the information system during the patients stay in hospital or on discharge. Other data are used for purposes of control of patient information and for communication with others about his location, basic religious faith, etc. All too often these important but non-medical aspects are overlooked but they are an essential part of patient care.

Clinical Data Module

The clinical data module contains several data segments and includes medical information about the patients present complaints, his present illness history in either normal or medical language. The past medical history usually deals with medical and surgical disorders and psychiatric and social difficulties of the past. A family history may be relevant if there are family or genetic factors related to the patients disorder or if the doctor thinks that 'risk factors' may be involved. There will be an occupational history telling the patients different occupations and a social history relating to housing and social relationships and activities. Other relevant histories may include a psychological history, an environmental history, a dietary history, a review of immunisation and vaccination, etc. The basic data to be entered into each of the segments should be defined and agreed between all those who enter the data into the medical information system.

For certain types of patient and in some hospitals, some or most of the historical information may be obtained from the patient directly. Such devices as questionnaires can provide responses to questions and give data to be entered into the information system. They are usually oriented to special disorders or may relate to general medical or surgical surveys. It is possible to obtain data from patients using devices such as a visual display unit or voice carrying system or taped questionnaire which can ask questions to which the patient responds and in this way data is recorded. Not only serial questions may be asked but a branched logic system allows a more detailed scrutiny of areas of information to which the patient responds positively. Naturally such planned data gathering systems require the design of objectives and must be patient-acceptable. There must always be a human system in reserve to support such questionnaire processing when necessary.

The next segment is that which deals with the physical examination of the patient, when abnormal structural or functional data will be observed by the doctor. These examinations may be recorded according to a fixed format or may be recorded as abnormal data where certain fixed examinations have taken place. Again such a segment has to have definite information objectives.

Both the information from the various relevant histories of the patients illness and the physical examination are used to reach a diagnosis or classification of the patients illness or problems. Usually a prognosis or predicted future for that individual patient is also derived from this data. The uses of these theoretical constructs are not only for administration purposes but to act as guides and controls for investigation and treatment of a patients disease or diseases.

Further information in some clinical data modules is derived from tests of body fluids such as urine, blood. This also forms input data to the diagnostic and prognostic module.

Diagnoses and Prognosis or Problem Module

Depending on the type of record system the basic theoretical constructs in this segment deal with either the formulation of working diagnoses or diagnostic hypotheses, or of problem definition in the Weed sense. It is important to clarify these two different approaches to defining the information content of this module.

The working diagnosis definition implies that these are diagnostic hypotheses, based on previous data which has to be explored and verified by patient investigation and the outcome of clinical management and treatment. These working diagnoses reflect the procedures of creating and proving scientific hypotheses which have been illustrated during the doctors basic training. On the other hand the Weed system defines the patient's problems, either from the point of view of the patient or the doctor. These problems are defined in terms of established states or abnormalities, which may exist at the time as an abnormal symptom or sign or as syndromes of diseases just as in the working diagnostic classification system. However, it must be emphasized that they are not hypotheses to be explored but defined and certain entities, which are later aggregated as problem definition proceeds.

The prognostic segment may relate to risk factors determined from the historical data and physical examination segments and is related to standard prognostic tables about survival rates in different diseases or related to the average life span of patients in general. There are several different ways to represent this type of information,some based on analyses of patients records and others based on information obtained from the medical literature. This information is linked to diagnoses.

It is important to recognise that no matter which formulation is used, it leads to the next module of progress notes or patient management data.

Patient Management Data or Progress Notes

There are at least three main segments in the module which relate to clinical state, investigation of working diagnosis or problems and therapy related to diagnosis or problem. This segment implies decisions about ordering these investigations and therapy in time and in relation to the importance of the information in both a positive and negative sense, since they will contribute to patient management.

In the decision-directed record, clinical decisions are recorded and the evidence which supported them in relation to investigative and therapy procedures. This allows for an audit trail to relate clinical decision to clinical outcome. In the problem-oriented record a different view is taken and the 'SOAP' logic is used to organise the data which related to plans which lead to the recording of subjective and objective data, assessment of this data, patient education and new plans for defining the patient's problems.

In the decision-directed record the clinical state forms a separate segment where information about symptoms and abnormal signs are recorded as frequently as the diagnosis and management requires. This information is used to monitor the effectiveness of treatment and also to produce information about changes in prognosis in response to management and treatment.

A fundamental process problem arises in these segments depending on whether investigative and therapy procedures are seen as orders from the medical team for certain activities and procedures to be carried out or are requests for investigation and treatment which have a different implication especially at the interfaces of request with process and subsystems. In the order procedure the doctor issues an order to the various investigative and therapeutic departments. They

carry out these orders in accordance with well defined procedures and
the doctor is given the result and acts accordingly, as he is
responsible for the interpretation of the results of his orders. For
example, this implies that a doctor may order a blood test such as
haemoglobin investigation or plasma electrolytes from the laboratory.
The results will be reported as the haemoglobin concentration for the
patient or the electrolyte values. The evaluation and interpretation
of this data will depend on the doctor who issed the orders and not
on the laboratory that carried them out.

In the request system there has to be a doctor-doctor interface for
the interpretation of both the process request and the result. Here
what is being requested is a scientific opinion from the doctor in
charge of investigation or therapy facilities. For example, if a chest
x-ray is wanted from a patient who is thought to have tuberculosis,
clinical data will have to be given with diagnostic information to
the doctor receiving the request. He may have other x-rays done than
those requested if he thinks they will better define the patients
diagnosis. The report of the x-rays of chest is a clinical opinion
from the radiologist based on both radiological and clinical data.
This is essentially a consultation system and leads to very different
processes from an order system.

Both an order and request system are used in investigative and
therapy activities in relation to patient management procedures. This
naturally relates to the type of input required for such processes for
it will vary not only with the request or order made but whether a
medical opinion has been sought about the result which will relate it
to previous clinical information. A more detailed discussion is not
appropriate at this time but the significance of the difference
arises from the different use not only of input information but of
ways of interpreting the output and modes of obtaining the data.

Discharge Module

This module has four main segments drawing together the results of the
activities both in investigation and treatment. Hopefully the patient
has recovered sufficiently for transfer to convalescence or to his
own home. He may require further treatment in another hospital. The
first segment deals with the final diagnosis and prognosis, the
prognosis of the patients recovery to date and his anticipated
prognosis when he leaves the hospital. The final diagnosis is the
diagnostic conclusion of the hospital care team and is used not only
for clinical but administrative classificatory purposes. Similarly,

in the Weed type medical record there would be a final list of active
and inactive problems. These statements provide the basis for future
medical action and continued treatment if necessary.

The discharge management segment deals with those management details
that ensure the patient will receive appropriate convalescence and
treatment, if necessary, when he leaves the hospital. It is important
that the treatment he has been given be communicated to the general
practitioner or other doctors who will care for him when he leaves
the hospital either in his home or in a convalescent hospital.

The hospital clinical summary segment draws together the important
features of the patients data obtained about his illness to guide the
future management of his illness or to provide an information base
for future care if this becomes necessary. It is essentially a summary
of existing recorded data and usually contains only abnormal results
and important features of the individual patients illness. It also
should clearly state the final diagnosis and prognosis and future
management decisions.

Other communication summaries of clinical data will be created
automatically or by the health care team for the general practitioner
or other doctors who will be responsible for the care of the patient
in future. The hospital summary and the summary for the general
practitioner may be similar but they usually express different views
of the patient data and hence are considered as separate segments.

Accounting and Audit Module

At the end of the stay of any patient in hospital it is necessary for
the health care team to briefly review the course and management of
that patients illness and some account should be taken in checking
that the management was optimal. Also there should be a patient view
of the functions of the clinical, nursing and other facilities so
that any problems met can be considered. Finally there should be a
segment which deals with cost-centred accounting procedures to
determine the cost of all resources deployed during the patients stay
in hospital. This completes the review process of a hospital episode
of illness of a patient. This view of accounting has been elaborated
in the decision-directed record.

The segment dealing with the patient's view of the functions of the
medical, nursing and other paramedical functions is important and is
usually determined by a standard questionnaire. It is designed not
only to allow criticism of the various things that may happen to the

patient but also so that he can give credit to the services which he has appreciated. This takes into account an important aspect of the morale of the caring team, who need some recognition of the utility of their activities.

The segment dealing with medical audit reviews the effectiveness either of the working diagnoses or of the problem list. It considers the changes brought about in the prognosis of the patient and reviews clinical management, especially the investigative pathway. The various aspects of treatment are also reviewed in the standard manner. This review is available for consideration at a later date should further review be considered.

The final segment deals with cost-centred accounting procedures. All that happens to the patient including medical and nursing activities, his hotel stay costs, the costs of investigation and treatment are obtained from the various segments of the record and a virtual cost determined for that patient. This will relate to the various elements of the cost, for example, the cost of investigation in laboratories and the costs of treatment facilities. It is, of course, the major cost centre in the hospital as the facilities are related to the clinical decision network about the patient. Most, if not all, the costing can be derived automatically from recorded data about the patient by a program. It is also possible to have running costs when the health care team consider it necessary. At present this study is in its initial phase.

Rehabilitation Module

This describes the patient's path of recovery, including convalescence and retraining for ordinary life. In describing the inpatient modules of the medical information systems, an attempt has been made to define the various modules of this system which reflect conventional and different aspects of the care process. Naturally, the importance and uses of each module vary with different disorders that are treated. Each module does deal with some aspect of patient care during an episode of illness and needs to be considered in any information system.

What is generally not recognised is that the progress notes or patient management module is by far the biggest part of the computer record in contrast with the traditional written record. Because of the accounting procedures for orders or requests it is necessary to have precise detailed records so that audit trails can be established.

The wealth of detail to cover the several purposes means that it is
necessary to have computer analysis of parts of the record and not to
try to review the whole record when printed out because of the wealth
of detail. This stresses that it is important to recognise that with
new tools there are new ways of dealing with information, for it is
possible to change the relationships between what is entered and what
is required by the users. These type of records add new dimensions
to medicine at some increased cost in the time spent by the health
care personnel who have to enter the data of the order of 20% to 30%.
However, it stops a great deal of time which is spent trying to make
the patient communication system and the information system work
under the existing situation plus a great number of telephone calls,
personal messages, etc. which are no longer necessary. We have not
reached the ideal medical record yet, but it is now possible for an
experimental approach to be used here to continue to improve patient
information systems.

References

1. de Heaulme, M., Anderson, J.: Medical record objectives in relation
   to clinical problems and user needs. Med. Informatics 3 (1978)
   37-50.

2. Jeanty, C.: The computerized medical record in gastroenterology.

   Part 1: Medical history-taking using questionnaires.
           Acta gastro-ent.belg. 39 (1976) 115-130;
   Part 2: Morphological (descriptive) data.
           Med. Informatics 3 (1978) 283-289;
   Part 3: Numerical laboratory data.
           Med. Informatics 3 (1978) 291-297;
   Part 4: Health curriculum vitae.
           Med. Informatics 3 (1978) 299-303.

3. Reichertz, P.L., Anderson, J.: A System view of Health Care
   Organizations. M. Laudet, J. Anderson, F. Begon (Eds.): Medical
   Computing, pp. 87-98. Taylor & Francis, London 1977.

4. Weed, L.L.: Medical Records, medical education and patient care:
   The Problem Oriented Record as a basic tool. Care Western Reserve
   Press Cleveland, 1969.

The Importance of 'Regionalisation' on the

Provision of Health Care

J.M. Forsythe

The dictionary definition of a region is an area, space or place of
more or less definite extent or character. The term regionalism
which it is derived from is the practice of regional systems or
methods.

Within the health delivery system its application is used to
identify some ordering or re-ordering of health resources and
services within an area. The concept can be viewed in two distinct
ways. The first, a top down approach, relates particularly to
nationalised systems of care, and represents a form of devolution
or the decentralisation of decision-making from the national
centre - whether it be government or otherwise - outward to a
number of areas within a nation. The importance of this within
health care cannot be over-emphasised. The correct balance of care
as between hospital and community health services or between
primary, secondary or tertiary prevention for a particular
community is something which must vary throughout any country. It
will be related to characteristics of the community such as its
age structure, cultural characteristics, family structures, social
class distribution, quality of housing, types of occupation and
opportunities for employment, environmental features and a great
deal more. In addition most democratic societies have realised
that within the health services the local consumers and providers
must have an important participative role in the planning of the
quantity and type of service. In Finland they identify this as an
inductive as against a deductive role. Of course in countries such
as mine,where the finance for health care tends to come from
central government, there must always be a system of accountability
from the periphery to the centre.

The second way in which regionalism is applied in health care represents a coalescence of neighbouring communities, institutions, agencies or programmes with a common interest. They band together to achieve progress which each member could not achieve alone. A centre or service is established to provide the entire periphery with services which otherwise would not be feasible, effective or economical. This represents rationalisation. It is an unfortunate fact of life that most people equate rationalisation with rationing but there is a world of difference between them as far as it affects both consumers and providers. Rationing means a fixed allowance or share of provisions, whereas rationalisation is the act of making rational and intelligible, and is a term which should be associated with improvement and advancement rather than restriction of a service. Taken as a whole it would achieve better access to care, improved quality of services, lower costs, greater equity.

Development of Regionalism within the United Kingdom

Because I can only claim real knowledge about the system of health care within my own country, I should like to trace the development of health regionalism. I have gone back as far as sixty years because, strangely enough it was in 1919 that the most important strategic document on the delivery of health care was produced in our country. It is as relevant today as it was then, and I believe its relevance is not just restricted to the United Kingdom, but exists everywhere else. The Report mentioned was called the Dawson Report (1). The terms of reference were "to consider and make recommendations as to the scheme or schemes requisite for the systematised provision of such forms of medical and allied services as should be available for the inhabitants of a given area".

I was amazed, not only to find in recent visits to the United States and Finland that this report was being quoted, but the whole text has recently been reproduced in the United States Milbank Foundation publication entitled "The Regionalisation of Personal Health Services" (2). The Dawson Report's recommendations for change were based on the fact that the organisation of medicine has become what it called 'insufficient' and because it fails to bring the advantages of medical knowledge adequately within reach of the people. The Report identified three levels of care which are clearly hierarchical. The Primary Health Centre embraces both preventive and curative medicine to a population through general practitioners, primary care doctors or dentists, nurses, midwives and supporting services such as health education, foot care, child health and school health clinics and selective screening. Care or preventive services would be given either at home or at the health centre which would also have beds available either on site or nearby for appropriate cases. Specialists would visit the Health Centre. The Secondary Health Centre was a place staffed by specialists where difficult cases or cases requiring special diagnostic facilities treatment would be referred from the Primary Centre. Finally, there are the Teaching Hospitals with medical schools which would act firstly as a secondary health centre for a designated area of primary health centres and, secondly, as a "tertiary" centre for dealing with cases of unusual difficulty and those requiring specialised knowledge or equipment referred from the secondary health centres. Such centres would also ensure the close interaction of teaching, research and service. It is perhaps worth noting that such a pattern of service is rational from the patients' point of view as well as for the providers. For those conditions which have a high probability of affecting each of us several times in a lifetime, e.g., respiratory diseases, musculoskeletal disorders, emotional problems or preventive measures, the primary health centre is appropriate. For more serious problems such as fractures, abdominal surgery or coronaries, which are less common, the secondary health centres are appropriate and, finally, there are the uncommon conditions requiring the highest level of knowledge, technology and facilities, which would be cared for in the tertiary centres.

The District General Hospital or Secondary Health Centre

The development of single specialty hospitals had been a notable feature of both voluntary and local government hospitals until the 1930's within the United Kingdom. We had separate hospitals, for example for maternity, eyes, ear nose and throat, orthopaedics, diseases of women, as well as those hospitals which were built to isolate patients from their community, e.g., for infectious diseases, tuberculosis, mental illness and mental handicap. It was the realisation that the geographical separation of specialties had become inappropriate which led to the development of what has today been called district general hospitals or secondary health centres. A beneficial byproduct of the second world war in England was the construction of what were called emergency medical service hospitals

which provided all the common acute hospital services for a
population on a single campus. These provided a wonderful pilot
scheme for the future district general hospitals.

The National Health Service

The introduction of the National Health Service in 1948 provided an
organisational framework which allowed the management of groups of
hospitals, previously under different ownership, to come under one
management committee. Thus one hospital management committee might
control up to twenty or more different hospitals, many of which were
single specialty. The country was divided into 14 Regions each with
up to five million inhabitants for overall planning of the hospital
services. Each Region had at least one undergraduate medical school.

Because of severe financial problems it was not possible to build
new hospitals until the early 1960's. In 1962, however, the
government introduced a hospital plan which identified the district
general hospital concept for the first time. Such a hospital was to
provide 600-800 beds and serve 100,000 - 150,000 population. Most
were to contain provision for all the ordinary acute specialties,
i.e., general surgery, medicine, paediatric, maternity, gynaecology
and orthopaedics. In addition there would be an emergency department
and the full range of out-patient services to deal with referrals
from doctors in primary care. There would also be full supporting
services from pathology, x-ray and rehabilitation departments. Some
acute beds would also be provided for psychiatry and geriatrics,
and there would also be beds primarily for cases needing nursing
care associated with the primary health centre. Beds for what might
be called 'super specialties' would only be provided in selected
hospitals, e.g. cardiothoracic surgery, neurosurgery. Because the
country had been divided up into 14 Regions, each of them would aim
to make itself self-sufficient for these specialties, although it
should be emphasised here there is no restriction as to which
specialist a patient might be referred to, so that patients could be
transferred to a hospital within a different region from their own.
All consultants were employed by the Regional Hospital Board except
in the undergraduate teaching hospitals and certain selected
postgraduate hospitals. It is obvious that it is essential to have
control of the number and location of specialists if there is to be
a rational provision of service.

The development under strict manpower control of training posts for specialty training within each region with linkage through rotation between the undergraduate teaching hospitals and the peripheral district general hospitals, and the secondment of medical students to peripheral hospitals, all helped to integrate the service, since the majority of medical students tend to take up career posts around their undergraduate teaching hospital – this helped to establish a lasting relationship in relation to patient referrals.

The construction of district general hospitals began in earnest in the late 60's. However, increased specialisation and the development of expensive technology raised the question as to whether the catchment or medical service area for a district general hospital of 100,000 – 150,000 was adequate. If one attempted to maintain the principle of one specialist working in isolation, and if one was going to provide services such as urology, paediatric surgery, endocrinology, nephrology or rheumatology on a district basis, then if the 100,000 – 150,000 medical service or catchment area was maintained, there would be insufficient numbers of specialists or finance for their supporting equipment to cover every district in the country. In 1969 a report (3) was introduced which recommended that in addition to the normal district specialties there should also be in every district the following specialties:

- Cardiology
- Thoracic Medicine
- Gastro-enterology
- Endocrinology
- Nephrology
- Communicable diseases
- Rheumatology
- Paediatric Surgery
- Thoracic (non-cardiac) surgery
- Peripheral Vascular Surgery
- Urology

The report recommended that, in order to achieve this with at least two specialists in each specialty, the size of a district general hospital should be increased so that it served 200,000 – 300,000 people. This meant that, if one included beds for the mentally ill and the elderly, the hospitals would all be at least 1,000 beds.

Big isn't Beautiful

It was about the early 70's that there were signs from work done
both in England and overseas that a hospital could be too big. Large
hospitals on one site may make accessibility difficult for some of
the population they are meant to serve, but even more worrying were
the problems of internal communications within the hospital with its
associated problems of staff morale and recruitment. A second
problem was that the rational provision of services for such things
as C.S.S.D. (Central Sterile Supply Department), laundries, certain
laboratory investigations, sterile fluid manufacturing, meant that
such services should be provided on a multidistrict and, in some
cases, a regional basis. However, in these services also the
original assumptions on which the cost-effectiveness of their size
were calculated have changed, particularly through the costs of
transport. There is no doubt, however, that quality control has been
improved. Within our country, however, there are dangers in over-
centralisation, particularly now that industrial action in the
health services is a harsh fact of life. The devastating effect of
the closure of a laundry serving 40-50 hospitals or a C.S.S.D.
serving half a region have only to be experienced once, in order to
make one realise that one mustn't put all one's eggs in one basket.
A third factor which has altered our thinking has been the
increasing development of consumer involvement in decision-making, -
some people might call this the democratisation of our health
service. The development of the new district general hospitals
inevitably means closure of existing units. If this involves a
particular hospital which has been built out of local philanthropy
and part of a community life over many years, it is hardly
surprising that there is some resistance to its closure,
particularly if it means the majority of the population will have
to travel further to the new facility. The development of what we
call 'community care' rather than 'hospital care' for the elderly
mentally ill and mentally handicapped has helped to increase the
public's interest and awareness of priorities within the health care
field. Day surgery and day hospitals have also been developing
rapidly.

We have had a significant change in policy against the large
district hospital. We are now thinking back to a population of
100,000 - 150,000 for a district hospital and, with our bed norms,
the size of the hospital will be around 600 beds. Such a hospital
will be supported by community hospitals situated in 'local

communities' and containing patients under the care of the primary
care physicians and with visits from local specialists for outpatient
referrals.

Increased Specialisation

There has been a tremendous increase in specialisation. There are
now 46 different specialties recognised today in England as against
the 22 in 1948. Many of the newer specialties do not normally see
patients referred by the primary care team but rather secondary
referrals from consultants, e.g., neuro-opthalmologist or neuro-
otologist, neonatal cardiac surgery, immunologists, transplant
surgeons. Clearly such people will function in 'tertiary care
centres', usually undergraduate teaching hospitals. It is important,
and our present system allows for this, that such people are not
involved in dealing with health care problems which could be more
easily dealt with by less specialised persons. In many countries
this happens because of the inadequate income the physician would
receive if he restricted himself to his narrow field. The dangers,
of course, are obvious,particularly when you see, for example,
cardiac surgeons only doing a dozen or so open-heart operations
annually. Although there had been a good deal of integration between
primary and secondary and tertiary care, it was still felt that our
organisational structure with the management and regionalisation
of the hospitals, but not of the other services, did not allow for
full integration.

In 1974 the N.H.S. in Britain was reorganised in order to achieve
a greater integration of the hospitals with primary care and other
community services,mainly preventative,which might be called the
regionalisation of comprehensive services. The pattern of referral
has not changed at all and the further development of the principles
contained within the Dawson Report is made easier.

The Benefits of a Regional Structure

What has been the main benefit from regionalisation of services?
The quality of care has been kept at a high level. Regional Health
Authorities are responsible for the appointment and location of
specialists. They are also responsible for the financing of
expensive equipment both medical and non-medical and the construction
of new buildings. It is possible,therefore,to ensure not only that
a new service is viable, but that one does not duplicate expensive

equipment and personnel. We hope, therefore, to ensure that there is a rational provision of services with equal access. As an example let me take open cardiac surgery and the development of cardiac pacemaker work. By getting together the specialists concerned, it was possible to reach agreement on the number of centres where such work would be performed. We have just agreed to reduce our cardiac surgical centres from four to three within my Region, and each Unit will perform between 300 - 500 open heart operations. Paediatric heart surgery will only be done in one of the three centres. Primary pacemaker insertion will only be done in three centres. Each of these centres will have at least two cardiac surgeons and two cardiologists.

It is important to realise that some services may start on a regional basis, but as the technology develops the service may develop to one which is available on a district basis, e.g., ultrasonic services for obstetrics or alpha-feto-protein serum estimator for screening in pregnancy.

Conversely, some services may change from a district or local service to a regional one. An example of this is intensive special care baby units for the newborn. Until recently we planned that each specialist obstetric unit would have a special care baby unit for low birth weight or sick neonates. We have now decided that there are a small number of neonates who are so sick that 'intensive' special care baby units should be available. Initially we have designated one such unit in the Region, but we plan to have three or four eventually. Special neonatologists will be appointed to each.

My own region also provides some services on a supra-regional basis, as do other regions. We maintain a national corneal bank for corneal grafts and we have a specialised renal dialysis unit for children, and a liver dialysis unit.

Finally, may I repeat that the United Kingdom model is not one I am trying to sell here today, but the concept of "regionalisation" is one which is necessary for every country, other than the smallest, as being one which ensures equal access, good quality care, good value for money, and yet allows some flexibility.

194

References

1. Interim Report on the Future Provision of Medical and Allied
   Services. Command. 693. Ministry of Health, London 1920.

2. Saward, F. (Edit.): The Regionalisation of Personal Health
   Services. Published for Milbank Memorial Fund by Prodist,
   New York 1975.

3. Central Health Services Council: The Functions of the District
   General Hospital. H.M.S.O., London 1969.

Use of Mortality, Morbidity and Risk Factors

in Epidemiological Models

M. Goldberg, M. Blanc, P. Le Beux,

P. Goldberg, F. Grémy

I. Introduction

The domain of public health is now one of the major public concerns
in industrialized as well as in less developed countries. The main
reasons for this are the ever rising costs of health care, the
technical and political difficulties in allocating scarce resources
between the different social sectors - education environment
control and so forth, health being only one of these sectors - and
the great complexity of the health care system, where one can
always find a great number of parameters interfering with each
other, most of them being poorly known and controlled, even in the
smallest subsystems such as, for instance, a hospital department.

While facing these difficulties bodies in charge of the health of
a population have, nevertheless, to make decisions: they must be
able to assess, predict, decide, allocate resources, control and
evaluate. Health planning is a necessity at the national, regional
or local levels, and,at each level, all the pertinent parameters
have to be taken into account and integrated in such a way that
the ultimate objective of the health system,namely to increase the
health level of the population,can be attained as effectively as
possible.

While the importance of health planning cannot be overestimated,
the relevant methodology is still underdeveloped, and there is a
great need for new tools.

The main basis of health planning techniques is the compilation
of vital and health statistics. It is a well known fact that, in
many respects, these statistics are insufficient: (1) their
quality is often very disputable, due to lack of motivation and/or
competence of the people collecting them in the field, (2) the

available data have often been chosen rather because of the ease
of collection than for their usefulness for health planning, (3)
the analysis techniques are still in progress: very likely, the
multidimensional techniques called "data analysis" (analyse des
données) are more efficient tools than classical Fisherian
methods. But we still remain in great demand of techniques able
to deal with evolutive data.

Mathematical modelling is still in its infancy. But the first
approaches are very promising (Kaihara, Klementiev, and the work
done at IIASA [1-4]). They seem useful for the following reasons:

- it is very difficult to make good and carefully planned
  experiments in the field of health care,

- the health care systems - and even health care subsystems -
  are very complex, due to the great number of factors involved.
  And there very rarely exists a one-to-one relationship between
  cause and effect. The alteration of one factor may often
  have other consequences than those obvious and expected.

- one of the sections of the mathematical modelling - called
  "system dynamics" - is especially aimed at describing and
  simulating dynamic phenomena (as opposed to purely statistical
  methods).

- even if the models remain purely theoretical, they can lead
  to better understanding and synthesis of health phenomena.

- as quoted, they can be useful tools for orienting subsequent
  epidemiological research (e.g., collecting useful and pertinent
  data).

- they may also allow to avoid difficult and expensive surveys
  by providing sufficient estimation of health indicators.

The present work deals
    (1) with an application of the model of A.A. Klementiev,
    (2) with the development and sophistication of this model.

II. The Model

Klementiev's model deals with degenerative diseases which are
closely connected with the aging process and which modifiy the
life expectancy of patients (e.g., C.V.D. and malignant tumors).
It is a morbidity model: the title of Klementiev's paper is

"On the Estimation of Morbidity", i.e. prevalence and incidence
of the diseases of interest [4].
It is composed of two submodels:
(1) a classical demographic submodel which gives the demographic
    projection by sex and age, if we apply to a given population
    definite laws of mortality, fertility and migration.
(2) An epidemiological submodel which implies the assumption of
    absence of recovery from the given disease (the corrected
    survival curves are supposed to be asymptotic to zero, as
    time increases).

Klementiev's epidemiological submodel is conceptually very
simple and shown dynamically in Figure 1.

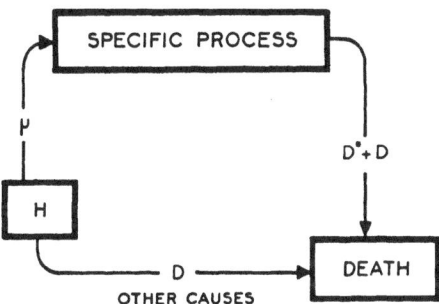

Fig. 1: Klementiev's epidemiologic sub-model for a degenerative
         disease.

The individuals are considered healthy if they are free from the
specific disease.

The healthy population will die either from the specific disease
under study or from other causes. μ, D and D* represent the
rates of exchange between the three possible states (μ = incidence,
D = general mortality rate, D* = specific mortality).

The model permits computing from usually available health and
demographic data the incidence and prevalence of the degenerative
diseases for every age and sex.

These data are (a) general mortality, (b) specific mortality and survival curves (Figure 2).

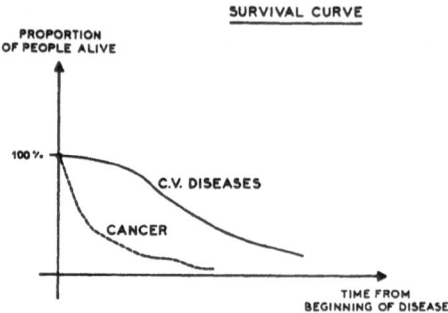

Fig. 2: Survival curves for C.V. diseases and cancers.

Figure 3 makes clear the general feature of the model:

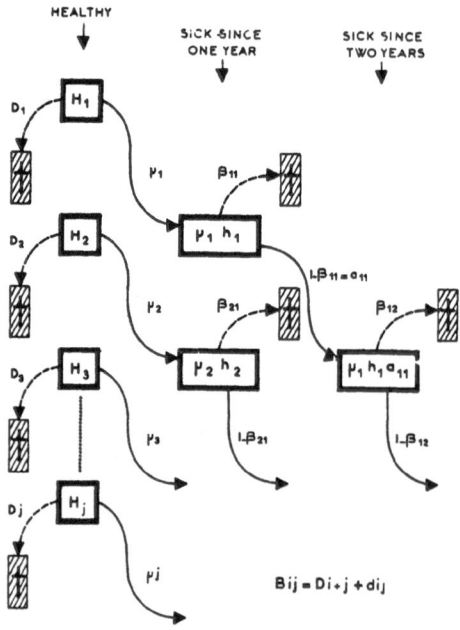

Fig. 3: Klementiev's epidemiologic and demographic model subdivided by years.

- h_1, h_2, ..., h_j represent the successive strata of the healthy population. The time which separates the strata is T_1 (usually one year).

- each stratum h_j may, during the time interval T, die from a "general" cause (mortality rate D_j) or contract the specific disease (incidence rate μ_j), or remain healthy.

- the terms $\mu_1 h_1$, $\mu_2 h_2$, ..., $\mu_j h_j$ represent people who have been sick since time T. They may die with a mortality rate β_{11}, β_{21}, ..., β_{j1} or survive with probability $a_{11} = 1 - \beta_{11}$, ..., $a_{j1} = 1 - \beta_{j1}$

- the terms $\mu_1 h_1 a_{11}$, $\mu_2 h_2 a_{21}$, ... represent people sick for two years, ... and so on.

In this graph, it becomes obvious that each row represents a stratum of the total living population; as for the columns, the hth column represents people sick since $(h - 1)T$.

Let us consider the β_{ij} coefficients; they are the total proportion of sick people aged i+j who die either from the specific disease, contracted j x T before, or from general causes. One can write

$$\beta_{ij} = d_{ij} + D_{i+j}$$

where D_{i+j} is the general mortality
      d_{ij} is the specific mortality rate for people who contracted the disease at age i and die at age i+j.

Obviously, the d_{ij} can be computed from the survival curves.
A first family of equations expresses that for every age and sex

Population = Healthy + Sick

$p_1 = h_1$

$p_2 = h_2 + \mu_1 h_1$

$p_3 = h_3 + \mu_2 h_2 + \mu_1 h_1 a_{11}$ $(a_{11} = 1 - \beta_{11})$

A second family of equations expresses that for every age and sex:

general mortality = specific mortality + mortality from other causes

$$p_1 \hat{D}_1 = h_1 D_1$$

$$p_2 \hat{D}_2 = h_2 D_2 + \mu_1 h_1 \beta_{11}$$

$$p_3 \hat{D}_3 = h_2 D_3 + \mu_2 h_2 \beta_{21} + \mu_1 h_1 a_{11} \beta_{12}$$

.

.

.

The general mortalities $\hat{D}_i$ are given by the demographic studies.
The "mortality causes" D_i are known if the mortality data D_i^* due to the specific diseases are available (usually through vital statistics):

$$D_i = \hat{D}_i - D_i^* .$$

Finally, if the following variables p_i, $\hat{D}_i$, D_i^* and the d_{ij} are known, it is possible to compute for every age and sex

h_i : number of healthy individuals

$\dfrac{p_i - h_i}{p_i}$: prevalence of the given disease

μ_i : incidence of the disease.

III. Application to the Evaluation of a Prevention Program

With such a model, it is possible to make several kinds of simulations. For instance, one can estimate the effects in the future which can be expected from an improvement of therapy, this factor intervening in the model through a modification of the survival curves.

One can also simulate the results of a preventive program. This is the topic of this presentation.

Usually, when evaluating the expected results of a prevention program aimed at the decrease of the incidence of a specific disease, one takes into account only this diminution, and makes the assumption that the individuals who have escaped the given disease go back to the healthy population. Reasoning in that way leads to an overestimation of the effects of the prevention program, because the other diseases are not taken into account. The effect of these other diseases on the population protected against the specific disease is a dual one:

(1) The specific disease is probably not stochastically independent of all the other diseases. This problem is quite complex and is far from being satisfactorily investigated. Recently, to better understand the interaction of several diseases, the concept of competing risk has been developed. This paper does not concern this problem and it is assumed that the specific and the other diseases are independent.

(2) The population protected against the specific disease gets older; after a certain age, the number of people in each age group will be greater than in the absence of an efficient preventive action. As the kind of disease which affects the population is very much age-dependent for the degenerative diseases, this phenomenon is observed through the specific mortality rates. The number of individuals who contract some other disease will be greater.

In order to solve this problem, we have used the model with two groups of diseases simultaneously: C.V.D. and cancer (Figure 4).

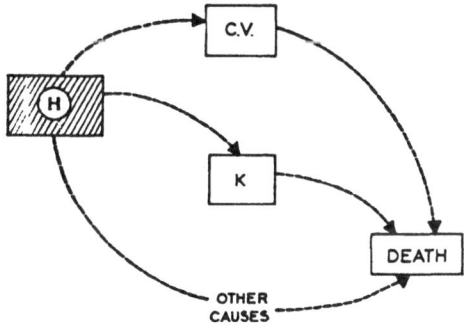

Fig. 4: Epidemiological model for two degenerative diseases: C.V. diseases and cancers.

We have taken the French population as given by the 1972 general census, and we assumed that the demographic laws will remain constant in the subsequent decades.

We adopted simple experimental curves for both groups of diseases, in the provisional absence of more precise data (mean survival time = 15 and 2 years respectively).

Then we decided on a scenario of prevention for C.V.D. leading to 50% reduction of specific mortality D_i^* between age 51-60. We did not assume any progress of therapy (survival curves unchanged)

In both situations - with and without preventive action - we have been able to compute for every age and sex the incidence and prevalence for both groups of diseases and to assess the results through 4 health indicators:

e_o : life expectancy at age 0

e_{40}: life expectancy at age 40

a : number of years of disease for 1,000 people

p : potential years of life lost for 1,000 people.

The main results are shown in Tables 1 and 2, devoted to C.V.D. and cancer respectively.

Years	e_o	e_{40}	a_{CV}	P_{CV}
0 (= 1972)	71.31	35.17	310	15.5
20	71.28	35.12	308	15.8
40	71.32	35.14	311	16.4

After preventive action against C.V. diseases

	e_o	e_{40}	a_{CV}	P_{CV}
0	71.51	35.39	293	14.0
20	71.48	35.34	290	14.2
40	71.52	35.35	290	14.5

Tab. 1: Health indicators before and after prevention for C.V. diseases: a_{cv} and P_{cv} concern the C.V. diseases.

Years	e_0	e_{40}	a_K	p_K
0 (= 1972)	71.31	35.17	17.02	15.39
20	71.28	35.12	17.44	16.00
40	71.32	35.14	18.25	16.67

After preventive action against
C.V. diseases

	e_0	e_{40}	a_K	p_K
0	71.51	35.39	17.09	15.39
20	71.48	35.34	17.65	16.06
40	71.52	35.35	18.33	16.74

Tab. 2: Health indicators before and after prevention for C.V.
diseases: a_K and p_K concern cancers.

It is possible to obtain the following results:

- increase of life expectancy e_0 and e_{40} (these figures are
obviously the same in both tables);

- decrease of a and p for C.V.D. (prevented disease) but less
and less effective in the long run;

- increase of a and p for cancer, more and more apparent
in the long run;

Keeping in mind that the initial data (survival curves) are
approximative and that some of the assumptions are rather crude
(constancy of demographic laws and of therapeutic effectiveness)
these results are shown just for their pedagogical value, but
one sees that the interaction exists. A model, fed with accurate
data, would allow to compute the gain and its evolution over
time. Such information can be of high value for health planners.

A possible criticism of <u>Klementiev's</u> model is the assumption of <u>absence of recovery</u>. But if the survival curve is asymptotic to a survival proportion (instead of zero), it presents no difficulty to write that a proportion α of sick people will die from other causes, and 1 - α from the disease of interest.

IV. Epidemiological Submodel for a Risk Factor

We have developed another submodel which is close to that of <u>Klementiev</u> in two respects:

- first, it is formally nearly identical,
- second, it deals with the way healthy people contract a given chronic disease after exposure to a given risk factor. As such, it is located upstream of <u>Klementiev's</u> submodel.

Our submodel is shown in Figure 5. The only formal difference with Klementiev's is the introduction of a flow which expresses the possiblity of coming back to healthy strata after a temporary exposure.

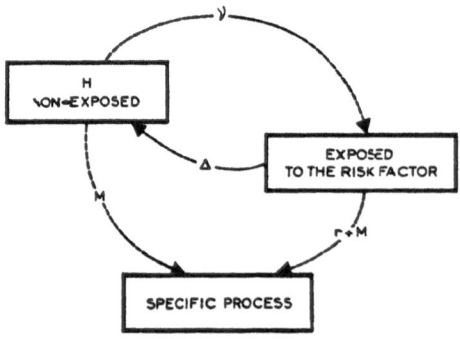

<u>Fig. 5</u>: Epidemiological model for a risk factor.

The matrix of Figure 6 divides the healthy population into
different categories: non-exposed, exposed 1 year, exposed 2
years, ...

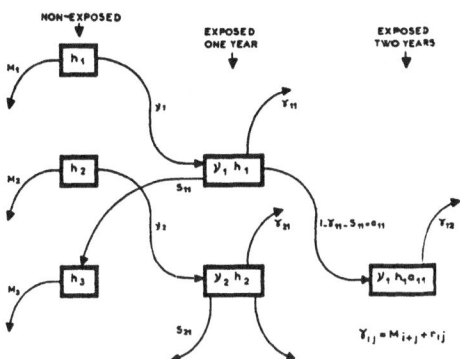

<u>Fig. 6</u>: Epidemiological model for a risk factor subdivided by years.

The M_i represents the incidence of the given disease for people
not exposed to the risk factor. In order to compute it, one must
know $\hat{M}_i$ "general specific incidence" (with and without exposure)
and M_i^* "specific incidence when exposed":

$$M_i = \hat{M}_i - M_i^* .$$

The ν_i are the "incidence" of the risk factor (i.e. the proportion of people who become, in a given period of time,
exposed to such a risk).

The S_{ij} are the proportion of individuals aged i+j who return
to complete health after an exposure of i years.

The γ_{ij} give the proportion of people aged i+j who fall ill
after exposure of i years.

These data could be obtained through the construction of
"resistance" curves, which are formally comparable to survival
curves: they indicate the proportion of individuals who have
not contracted the disease in relation to the duration of
exposure (Figure 7).

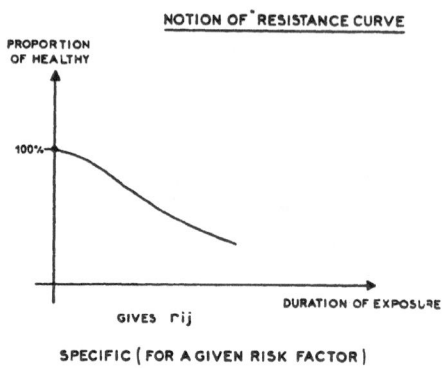

NOTION OF RESISTANCE CURVE

PROPORTION OF HEALTHY

100%

DURATION OF EXPOSURE

GIVES r_{ij}

SPECIFIC (FOR A GIVEN RISK FACTOR)
MORBIDITY RATE

Fig. 7:   Schema of a curve of resistance to a risk factor.

The equations are divided into two classes:

The first class expresses

> healthy = healthy non exposed + healthy exposed

$$H_1 = h_1$$
$$H_2 = h_2 + v_1 h_1$$
$$H_3 = h_3 + v_2 h_2 + v_1 h_1 s_1 + v_1 h_1 a_{11} \ldots$$

The second class expresses

> sick = sick after exposure + sick without exposure

$$H_1 M_1 = h_1 M_1$$
$$H_2 M_2 = h_2 M_2 + v_1 h_1 \dot{\gamma}_{11}$$
$$H_3 H_3 = h_3 M_3 + v_2 h_2 \gamma_{21} + \gamma_1 h_1 \gamma_{11} \gamma_{12}$$

One can notice that the H_i and the M_i can be computed from
Klementiev's model (they are the h_i and the v_i of the preceding
paragraph respectively).

The output of such a model is the computation of the "incidence" and "prevalence" of risk factors. The estimation of such parameters can be useful in two ways:

- theoretically, it could be used to assess exposure to a given risk factor, without having to undertake lenghthy and expensive surveys;

- by integrating the two models described (the risk model and Klementiev's model) into a "full model". Evaluation of prevention programs can become much more realistic, allowing to simulate programs intended to modify exposure to risk, expressed directly in terms of results (e.g. decrease in mortality).

For the time being, the model remains purely theoretical; in fact, the "resistance curves" are not accurately known. But the model motivates further research in order to obtain such data.

A weak point of the model is the S_{ij}: no data are available giving such information. Moreover, the S_{ij} do not cover a clear concept. It is very doubtful to pretend that, after a temporary exposure of i years without contracting the disease, an individual becomes a "healthy exposed", as soon as he ceases to be exposed.

References

1. Kaihara, S., Atsumi, K.: A system approach to Japanese medical care using a simulation model. Proceed. IIASA bio-med. Conf. Laxenburg, Austria, 1975.

2. Kaihara, S., Fujimasa, I., Atsumi, K., Klementiev, A.A.: An approach to building a universal health care model: morbidity model of degenerative diseases. Internat. Inst. Appl. Systems Analysis, Laxenburg, Austria, 1977.

3. Klementiev, A.A.: Mathematical approach to developing a simulation model of a health care system. RM - 76-55, IIASA, Laxenburg, Austria, 1976.

4. Klementiev, A.A.: On the estimation of morbidity. IIASA, Laxenburg, Austria, 1977.

The Structure of Physicians' Activities in General Practice and Modelling their Degree of Coverage*)

P.L. Reichertz, B. Schwarz, H.J. Meldau

The development of problems in health care delivery, both in regard to quality and quantity as well as the resulting economic repercussions, induces system analytical studies in various contexts. In reporting results of such projects one has to bear in mind the differences in the various health care delivery systems (24, 26, 27), which may vary in the basic structure and type of finance. Also, specific health care delivery systems induce specific problems, though all industrialized countries share the problem of an increasing economic load due to higher consumption or provision of health care services and the impact of technology.

Having a central position in the field of sociological and political interest, attempts to influence the behavior of the health care delivery system aim at two objectives which may conflict:

1) to improve the quality of health services, mostly under the rationale to arrive at optimal or at least equal accessibility for all and

2) to reduce the increasing cost while maintaining or even improving the quality of care.

*) This investigation was supported by a grant of the Robert Bosch-Stiftung, Stuttgart and in part by the 'Zentralinstitut für die Kassenärztliche Versorgung in der Bundesrepublik Deutschland', Cologne, Fed. Rep. of Germany.

To change systems, however, one needs in-depth knowledge of the controlling factors (24, 26, 27, 29). The difficulty of quality assessment is caused by the multivariate nature of subjective value scales entering each evaluation of a health care system. Nonetheless, indicators may be used under defined conditions of comparison as a measurement for the process (24, 27), not necessarily the result.

This should not be mistaken for a naive belief that these indicators

- reflect the actual state of a health care system and
- therefore, are absolute measurements of quality.

In political discussions, however, such indicators are often used and sometimes, either directly or indirectly, become the basis of legislative measures.

Thus legislature in the German Federal Republic requests a mandatory physicians' organization ('Kassenärztliche Vereinigung', KV) as an interface between physicians and the insurance system (respectively the sickness funds). Besides the administration of reimbursement claims from the health insurance system, it is the task of this organization "to guarantee primary medical coverage". The law, however, does not specify how this coverage should be measured. It has to be added that the German health system is the classical insurance system with mandatory insurance schemes. Local sickness funds are held by law to administer the funds collected from the participants and to regulate claims with the physicians' organization already mentioned. Patients do not pay directly but hand a claim cheque over to the physician, and the hospitals deal directly with these sickness funds on the basis of per diem rates. About 90-94% (21) of all ambulatory patients fall under this mandatory health plan, additional and voluntary private insurance being possible and used mostly for hospital care.

In order to fulfil the legal requirement to guarantee medical coverage, certain indicators have been investigated to serve as a basis for evaluation. Of all indicators, up till now, only the relation coefficient ('Masszahl') was maintained which indicates the number of people in a region per general practitioner. However, it has to be understood that practitioners differ very much in their spectrum of activities, number of cases treated and intensity of care (21, 25, 30). Specialists, too, participate in primary care delivery. The demand, on the other hand, may vary according to the density of the region, industrial structure, migration of workers into or out of the region, commuting, age structure, etc.

The objective of our investigation was to arrive at a dynamic model which reflects the determinant variables for the providers as well as the consumers and to study the effects of changes in population statistics including shift of age groups on both sides, structural changes, urbanization etc. in order to arrive at predictive values both for actual comparison and planning purposes.

The model was based on the data of the regional physicians' organization (KV Niedersachsen; (13)) as well as on the results of a structural analysis of approximately 2,000 general practices in Lower Saxony (28, 30).

Since the results of the structural analysis are of general interest in regard to analysis of health care delivery, some results will be described which are beyond the scope necessary for the construction of the model.

The original objective of the structural analysis (30) was to prove the hypothesis (25) that organizational and behavioral variables may be used to identify several types of general practices which as such offer different conditions for support by organizational means and EDP technology. The original objective was met, but the results obtained also yielded further insight into general problems. Using multivariate techniques, eight clusters of types of general practices could be identified with characteristic variables and behavioral aspects which allowed for predictions as to suitability for EDP support. Several factors of administrative, medical and financial components were identified and described. These results were tested against actual implementations of seven computers on a microprocessor basis in general and specialized practices which had been typed accordingly. The results of the grouping, though they will not be discussed in detail in this context, show very clearly that the element of general practice in health care delivery is not a uniform element but shows various types and dependencies which any detailed analysis or planning has to account for (31).

The analysis (30) is based on questionnaires mailed to the general practitioners and data available from the physicians' organization. Approximately 60% of the questionnaires were sent back and, after eliminating incomplete or dubious answers, a total of 56.3% of the total population could be covered.

The age distribution shows a strong emphasis on the age groups between 55-59 and 60-64 years. The retrieved sample differs only slightly from the distribution in the total population.

In the sample the mean age of physicians was 38 when opening the practice. This indicates a long activity in hospitals and tertiary care environments before starting the career of a general practitioner. Accordingly, older physicians prevail. However, in recent years a tendency can be seen to settle down in practice at an earlier age (30).

The number of paramedical people employed varied between 0 and 9, with an average value of 2.6 full-time equivalents also considering family members. Activities outside the physician's office are reflected in the number of house-calls per week. They had an average value of 43 and a median in the class between 41 and 50/week. It has to be noted that 2% indicated more than 100 house-calls/week.

The percentage of specific medical procedures varies and shows peaks in the area of "small"surgery, pediatrics and ear, nose and throat diseases. This indicates certain types of preferences, necessities and requirements for curriculum design and postgraduate education. The various results in regard to organizational factors, number of files, functions and layout of the doctor's office will not be discussed in this context (30). Of general interest is the distribution of turnover from revenues received under the mandatory insurance system. A slightly different distribution shows the number of patients treated per treatment period. (Within the German system, the insured person is treated for whatever disease and for any number of contacts on one single claim cheque which is valid for one quarter of a year. Such a patient is referred to in this context as case per treatment period. For details about number of contacts per case see 20 and 21).

Analyses were performed in regard to the location of practice.
Higher revenues are obtained in the rural areas (mainly due to
larger number of cases). Revenues and their relation to the number
of personnel were investigated.

TYPE OF PRACTICE	AVERAGE TURN-OVER	STANDARD DEVIATION	N
RURAL PRACTICE	221.000.2	± 108.633.4	588
SMALL TOWN	202.967.7	± 121.325.1	455
LARGE CITY	191.356.3	± 109.355.5	548
--------			-----------
TOTAL	200.776.5	± 113.272.7	1591

	AVERAGE TURN-OVER	STANDARD DEVIATION	N
SMALL LABORATORY	173.610.3	± 93.657.7	765
AVERAGE SIZE	239.209.6	± 111.697.8	699
LARGE LABORATORY	285.690.5	± 163.686.1	79

TOTAL	209.065.9	± 112.629.1	1543

Fig. 1: Average turnover/year according to the site of the
practice and a high or a low volume of laboratory
examinations (30).

Some results in regard to the influence of technology are of inter-
est.Offices with large laboratories showed an increase of revenues
by approximately 65% against those with only low laboratory
activities. The turnover per case is increased by 40 percent
approximately, thus the total increase is caused both by the number
of cases as well as by turnover per case. Taking those laboratories
which are described by the physicians in the sample as being large
in volume and applying objective measures as far as the spectrum of
analyses performed is concerned, a sub-sample of 64 was investigated. Here the difference between a small spectrum and a large
spectrum (both having a large volume of analyses) is 66%. In this
case, however, the turnover per treatment case only shows an increase
of roughly 10% in the laboratories with a large spectrum compared with
those having only a small one. Here the peak lies in   the laborato-

ries with a medium spectrum being 20% higher than the group with
a small spectrum and 9% higher than the group with a large spectrum.

"LARGE LABORATORIES ACCORDING TO SPECTRUM OF ANALYSIS"	TURNOVER	STANDARD DEVIATION	N
SMALL SPECTRUM	218,143 (206,963)	119,028.6 (110,784)	28 (26)
AVERAGE SPECTRUM	250,882 (250,121)	130,209.1 (139,048)	14 (12)
LARGE SPECTRUM	362,349 (362,349)	125,304.2 (125,304)	22 (22)
TOTAL	274,875 (272,569)	137,965.7 (139,279)	64 (60)

Fig. 2: Turnover/year in general practices in Lower Saxony
(30) in regard to the spectrum of laboratory analyses
performed. (In parenthesis those which do not belong
to group practices or laboratory sharing groups).

Of particular interest for the model were the age distributions.
According to the emphasis on higher age groups, the number of
treatment cases covered by the age groups between 56-60 and
61-65 years was highest.

However, when analyzing the individual throughput for the various
age groups, a decrease of treatment cases and revenues can be
clearly seen with increasing age. The same tendency prevails when
considering the time in practice.

NUMBER OF TREATED CASES (PATIENTS IN QUARTERLY TREATMENT PERIODS)
IN THE VARIOUS AGE GROUPS

AGE GROUP	NUMBER OF CASES/YEAR	N
→ 30	4 010	1
31 - 35	210 820	38
36 - 40	408 964	77
41 - 45	346 219	53
46 - 50	465 490	71
51 - 55	920 366	148
56 - 60	1 371 588	250
61 - 65	1 443 601	277
66 - 70	780 906	174
71 - 75	108 045	34
> 76	94 618	45
	6 154 627	1 168

Fig. 3: Distribution of age groups (n) and total number
of cases treated by this age group in
Lower Saxony (30).

The number of partnerships is still small in Germany. Laboratory
sharing prevails and occurs in approximately 19%.

73% of all general physicians do not belong to any type of loose
or closer partnership, which is only found in 2.9 - 5.3% of the
cases, considering the various possibilities legally feasible.

AGE CLASS	AVERAGE TURNOVER	STANDARD DEVIATION	N
31 - 35	238.889,1	± 112.101,8	51
36 - 40	228.971,3	± 145.612,9	129
41 - 45	275.259,6	± 130.705,0	84
46 - 50	252.095,0	± 122.948,1	99
51 - 55	235.805,4	± 124.007,9	216
56 - 60	214.770,1	± 93.934,9	344
61 - 65	191.758,1	± 93.676,6	364
66 - 70	165.385,2	± 91.485,3	213
71 - 75	132.349,9	± 78.799,4	40
MORE THAN 76 YEARS	76.948,2	± 63.700,0	50
TOTAL	206.778,3	± 113.282,1	1590

IN PRACTICE SINCE	AVERAGE TURNOVER	STANDARD DEVIATION	N
UNDER 6 YEARS	281.819,6	± 123.297,8	229
6 - 10 YEARS	246.503,8	± 134.414,1	142
11 - 15 YEARS	227.860,6	± 115.685,6	170
16 - 20 YEARS	237.803,3	± 105.782,8	273
21 - 25 YEARS	204.446,8	± 120.475,6	225
26 - 30 YEARS	187.519,4	± 87.211,5	358
31 - 35 YEARS	185.868,9	± 91.762,2	101
36 - 40 YEARS	175.170,3	± 109.737,1	53
41 - 45 YEARS	81.611,0	± 46.082,7	17
46 - 50 YEARS	70.915,5	± 46.082,7	11
MORE THAN 50 YEARS	62.578,7	± 80.015,3	12
TOTAL	206.778,1	± 113.282,6	1591

Fig. 4: Average turnover in general practice in
Lower Saxony (30) in regard to age of
physician and time in practice

In constructing the model, use was also made of time measurements in
a selected number of practices (20, 21, 25) and number of contacts/
case. The principal concept of the model was to calculate the
effective number of providers and setting this number in relation
to the effective number of inhabitants. Certainly, such an
approach is naive in terms of definition of the need and reflects
only actual demand, but it is, at the moment, the only method
effectively applicable for planning and determining the coverage
according to the legal requirements, lacking data and reliable

models for the prediction of incidence of conditions and their
translation into actual need versus demand. The model is meant to
be usable as such in the actual environment on available data. It
may, however, very well enter more comprehensive simulation
approaches adjusting the population of the suppliers and the
consumers. Under these constraints and simplifications, the model
tends to describe the process rather than the causes. It is designed
for application in a restricted and practical context.

The model basically adjusts the effective number of providers
according to the regional situation and structure of the providers
and relates this effective number of 'man units' or 'GP-equivalents'
in primary care to the adjusted ('effective') number of consumers.
The variables used to determine the adjustment of the providers
are:

- age structure of the physicians of the region
- their sex distribution
- number of treatment cases in the region
- percentage of partnership practices
- estimate of primary care provided by specialists
  in the region
- physician's time in general practice
- working hours
- average waiting time per contact
- location of practice (rural, small city, large city)
- number of auxiliary personnel
- number of house-calls
- size of laboratory
- degree of organization of practice
- postgraduate training
- spectrum of diagnostic assessment
- spectrum of procedures recorded
- time spent per patient
- participation in emergency services
- accessibility of practices.

The first five variables could be obtained for four test regions
which are also defined as unit of regional planning:

1) a metropolitan area (Braunschweig)
2) a suburban area bordering this metropolitan area (Sickte)
3) a small city and its environment (Gifhorn) and
4) a rural area (Hankensbüttel).

Some data were available from the physicians' organization (3, 13);
for other variables mean values were takén from the data of the
structural analysis (30). For some, regional averages were used.
The known age structure of the region was put into relation with the
average activities for the various age groups found in the structural
analysis, and adjustments were made in regard to working time
provided by women versus men. Analyses (16) had shown that 85% of
the female physicians worked more than 40 hrs/week compared to 94%
of their male colleagues. Adjustments for the percentage of primary
care provided by specialists were made according to the mix of
specialties in the region. Waiting time estimates were based on a
previous analysis in Lower Saxony (3, 21) according to the type of
region (metropolitan, suburban, small city and rural area).

In the same fashion, adjustments were made for the number of paramedical personnel, house-calls in the region, volume and spectrum
of laboratory, organizational structures and participation in emergency services. Previous studies had yielded information in regard
to the distribution of the various activities of the physicians
during the contact with the patient (20, 21).

The accessibility of the practice was evaluated according to an
algorithm given by (1):

$$Ds = \frac{\sum_{i=1}^{n} e_i \times E_i}{T_E} \times D$$

n: number of agglomerations in
   the region

e_i: distance of the i-th agglomeration
   to the next seat of a primary care
   physician

E_i: number of inhabitants of the region

T_E: total inhabitants of the region

D: density of population of the region

DS: distance to next seat of a primary
   care physician

Fig. 5: Algorithm to evaluate accessibility (according to 1).

This score, however, did not enter the model as such, but was calculated separately, since it could not yet be determined how it would
affect the degree of coverage. It is estimated that values larger

than 200 may indicate an insufficient degree of coverage. In the present samples, the score was between 100 and 170.

The effective number of providers was computed by determining the mean value of the various factors multiplied by the number of primary care physicians plus the primary care equivalent of the specialists in the region. Since some variables are of greater importance than others, weighting was performed in another equation giving greater emphasis to the factor of age and sex distribution, working hours, organization and number of cases.

$$GPE = NGP * \frac{\sum_{i=1}^{17} V_i}{17} + SPECE$$

GPE: effective rate of G.P.'s
NGP: normal rate of G.P.'s
V_i: variables of the i-th agglomeration
SPECE: specialists participating in primary care delivery

Fig. 6: Equation for the effective number of providers.

$$INH = T_i * \frac{\sum_{i=1}^{6} V_i}{6} + MIG$$

INH: inhabitants of the region
T_i: total inhabitants of the region of the i-th agglomeration
V_i: variables of the i-th agglomeration
MIG: migration of the region

Fig. 7: Equation for the determination of the effective number of consumers

The variables determining the demand (not the need) were considered to be the following:

- age of the population
- sex distribution
- educational structure
- accessibility to information
- style of living
- family situation
- employment rate
- mix of professions
- financial situation
- standard of living
- nationality
- population density
- percentage of commuters
- economic structure of the region
- degree of urbanization.

The underlined variables were implemented in the model and the data were read in according to demographic information available for the region. Then the number of inhabitants was adjusted in order to arrive at the effective number of consumers. The relation between the effective number of primary care physicians was then set in relation to the effective number of inhabitants to arrive at the corrected ratio.

The model (19) was written in CSMP (10) according to the principles described by Forrester (5). According to the suggestions of Klimke (15), the following feedback mechanisms were programmed:

- feedback between number of patients and overload of primary care physicians,

- feedback between number of physicians in primary care and their workload,

- feedback between number of providers and demand resp. number of cases,

- feedback between the number of hospital physicians going into primary care and attractivity of work in primary care.

The first feedback loop surmises that general practitioners are having an influence on the demand respectively the number of cases treated. Demand may be generated by more activity, less referrals and vice versa.

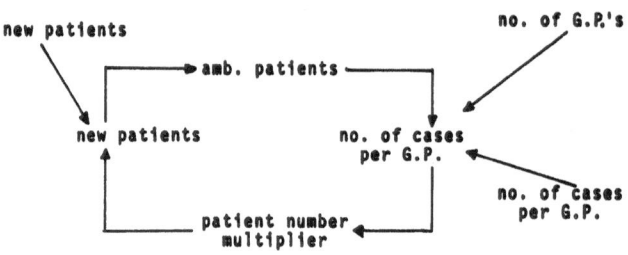

GENERATION OF DEMAND

Fig. 8: Feedback loop for the generation of demand based on the number of cases (according to 15)

The second loop describes the relation between demand and number of physicians: increase in number of cases increases the demand for new physicians in the region.

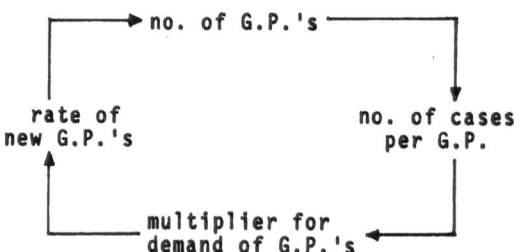

Fig. 9: Incentive for G.P.'s to settle in the area (according to 15)

The third loop indicates that the number of GP's in a region has an influence on the demand of the population.

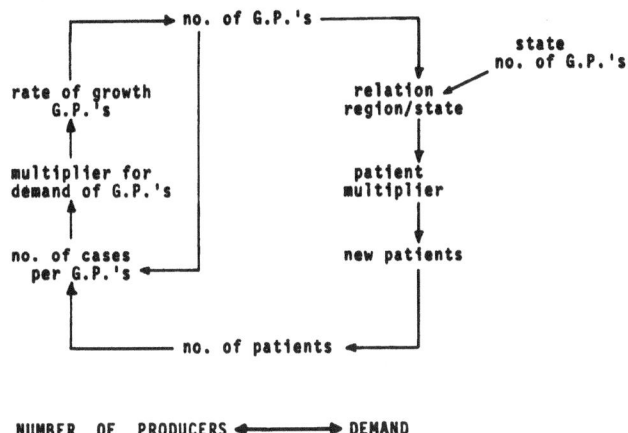

NUMBER OF PRODUCERS ◄──────► DEMAND

Fig. 10: Feedback loop describing the increased demand
generation by an increasing number of providers (15)

The fourth feedback loop describes the migration of hospital physicians into private practice and considers workload and resulting attractiveness as factors of the degree of migration.

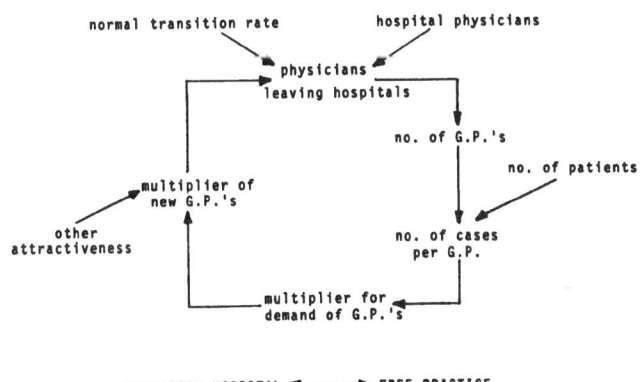

MIGRATION HOSPITAL ◄──────► FREE PRACTICE

Fig. 11: Migration of physicians from hospital positions
into private practice (15)

The two subsystems 'demand' and 'supply' of the model are constructed using these feedback loops.

222

The rates and basic data were taken from the structural analysis
(30) and various other statistical, demographical or analytical
publications (3, 9, 15, 16, 17, 22). Specific regional data were
obtained and supplied to the model. The time interval was chosen
to be one week over a period of five years. Population growth was
determined from changes in previous years: a growth rate of 1% was
assumed (18).

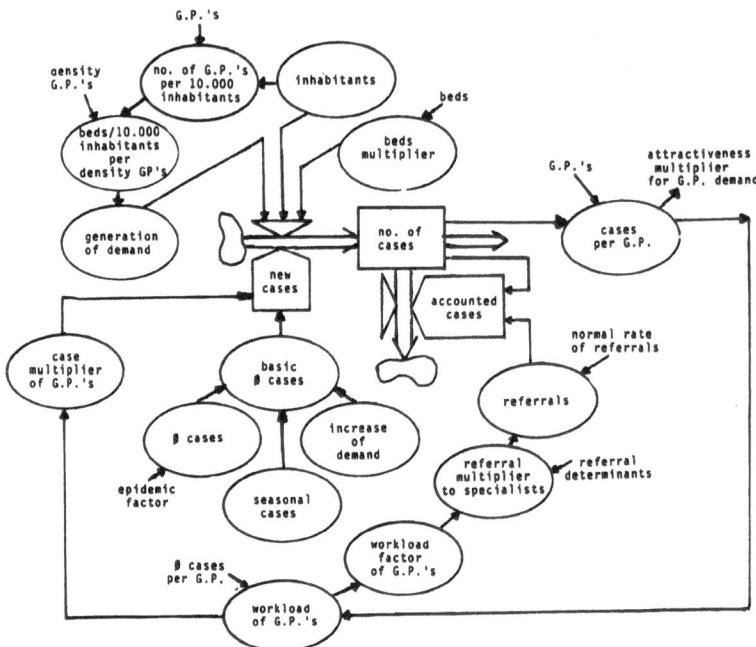

Fig. 12: Model of the subsystem 'demand' (according to 15)

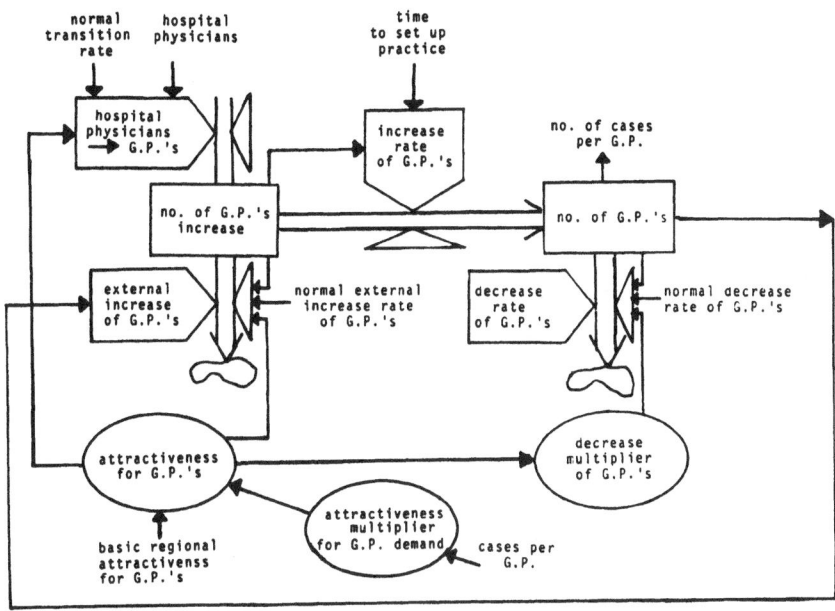

Fig. 13: Model of the subsystem 'supply' (according to 15.)

The simulation runs yielded different degrees of actual coverage and showed the prospective development in the tested regions.

The metropolitan area (Braunschweig) has many commuters and specialists. The overall degree of coverage was calculated to be high with 1,761 or 5.7 GP-equivalents for 10,000 'effective' inhabitants. The model predicts a decrease of coverage of 2.4% over the next five years. This will be the result of the age structure of the physicians in this region, the growing tendency towards specialization and the development of the population. The 'effective' population is considered to be 21% higher than the census population due to a high number of incoming commuters. A test run has been made to show the influence of the age structure of the physicians: A decrease of the average age by 2 years results in an estimated increase in the work capacity by one GP-equivalent which was approximately 1%.

The region (Sickte) bordering the metropolitan area (suburban area) showed the lowest degree of coverage of the four regions. Despite the great number of outgoing commuters it was calculated to be 2,576 respectively 3.9 GP-equivalents per 10,000 inhabitants and therefore beyond the value of 2,400 respectively 4.2 which is considered to be a critical value for beginning undercoverage.

This is also reflected in the high number of cases per GP. Due to changes in the structure of the area and the various inherent factors, the model predicts a further decrease of coverage by approximately 19% over the next five years.

The region of the small city (Gifhorn) has a similar degree of coverage as the large city: 1,739 respectively 5.7/10,000. This is the result of a great number of specialists with their respective primary care equivalents. The decrease of coverage will be the result of population increase versus a relatively constant effective number of GP's.

The best actual degree of coverage was found in the rural area (Hankensbuettel) reaching 1,596 or 6.3 GP-equivalents/10,000. Despite the high degree of coverage, the number of cases/GP is not below average, confirming the assumption of the first feedback loop. The model predicts a decrease of coverage by 23% over the next five years.

In simulation runs the overall factors to calculate the effective number of practitioners were between 0.964 and 0.996. For the inhabitants the factor varied between 1.0156 and 1.0739.

The model intends to be a tool for practical application and planning. Its time predictions will be tested in the various regions. The pessimistic predictions in regard to a decrease of coverage may be somehow corrected by a factor not yet implemented and reflecting the strongly increasing number of medical students over the last years. But there still is little tendency to go into private practice and planning efforts have to concentrate on the attractiveness of this career.

Though the ultimate goal is to develop models explaining the causal relationships in health care delivery (e.g. 6, 11, 14, 23) and their results, models describing a particular aspect of the process (e.g. 2, 4, 7, 8, 12) may be of practical value and ultimately will be the elements of more comprehensive efforts, when their validity has been proven.

The purpose of this model was to provide help in decision making in planning and assessment in a region, based on available data. It is our hope that, with further development and refinement of the model, the process of decision making may be guided towards the more essential issues of health care delivery such as to define need and develop models to match the resulting demand.

References

1. Beske, F.: Kassenärztliche Bedarfsplanung. Gutachten zum Entwurf eines Planungsansatzes für die Bedarfsplanung. Schriftenreihe des Zentralinstituts für die kassenärztliche Versorgung in der Bundesrepublik Deutschland, Heftreihe Bd. 9. (Deutscher Ärzteverlag, Köln 1977).

2. Bigelow, J.H., Brown, H.L.: Factors Affecting Participation in Cervical Cancer Screening Programs. (International Institute for Applied Systems Analysis, IIASA Publication RM-75-62, Laxenburg 1975).

3. Bossmann, A.: Praxis '72. Praxisanalyse der KV Niedersachsen. (Kassenärztliche Vereinigung Niedersachsen, Hannover 1972).

4. Fleissner, P.: Comparing Health Care Systems by Socio-Economic Accounting. (International Institute for Applied Systems Analysis, IIASA Publication RM-76-19, Laxenburg 1976).

5. Forrester, J.W.: Industrial Dynamics - After the First Decade. Mngmt Sci. 14 (1968) 398-415.

6. Fujimasa, I., Kaihara, S., Atsumi, K.: A Morbidity Submodel of Infectious Diseases. (International Institute for Applied Systems Analysis, IIASA Publication RM-78-10, Laxenburg 1978).

7. Gibbs, R.J.: Health Care Resource Allocation Models - A Critical Review. (International Institute for Applied Systems Analysis, IIASA Publication RM-77-53, Laxenburg 1977).

8. Gibbs, R.J.: A Disaggregated Health Care Resource Allocation Model. (International Institute for Applied Systems Analysis, IIASA Publication RM-78-1, Laxenburg 1978).

9. Häussler, S.: Praktischer Arzt - Facharzt - Klinik. Krankenhausarzt 41 (1968) 241-243.

10. IBM: System/360 Continuous Modelling Program - User Manual. IBM Program No. 360A-CX-16X.

11. Kaihara, S., Fujimasa, I., Atsumi, K., Klementiev, A.: An Approach to Building a Universal Health Care Model: Morbidity Model of Degenerative Diseases. (International Institute for Applied Systems Analysis, IIASA Publication RM-77-6, Laxenburg 1977).

12. Kaihara, S., Kawamura, N., Atsumi, K., Fujimasa, I.: Analysis and Future Estimation of Medical Demands Using a Health Care Simulation Model: A Case Study of Japan. (International Institute for Applied Systems Analysis, IIASA Publication RM-78-3, Laxenburg 1978).

13. Kassenärztliche Vereinigung Niedersachsen: Kassenärztliche Versorgung in Niedersachsen - Strukturanalyse der KV Niedersachsen Hannover (1977).

14. Kiseleva, G.: The Influence of Urbanization on the Birthrate and Mortality Rate in Major Cities of the USSR. (International Institute for Applied Systems Analysis, IIASA Publication RM-75-68, Laxenburg 1975).

15. Klimke, W.A.: Dynamische Systemanalyse der ambulanten und stationären Krankenversorgung einer Region. In: Wahl, M. (Hrsg.): Wiss. Beiträge Karlsruhe (Verlag Wahl, Karlsruhe 1976).

16. Koller, S.: Ärzteanalyse: Zahl, Struktur und Nachwuchsbedarf der Ärzte. Ergebnisse der Volks- und Berufszählung 1961, ergänzt auf den Stand 1967. (Bundesministerium für Jugend, Familie und Gesundheit, Bonn 1970).

17. Lüth, P.: Niederlassung und Praxis. (G. Thieme Verlag, Stuttgart 1969).

18. McKinsey & Co., Inc.: Hochschulabsolventen im Beruf. Ausbildungs-
    bedarf für Mediziner bis zum Jahr 2000. Bundesministerium für
    Bildung und Wissenschaft (Hrsg.). (Gersbach, München 1974).

19. Meldau, H.J.: Entwicklung eines deskriptiven Modells für die
    ambulante ärztliche Versorgung. (Diplomarbeit, Techn. Univ.
    Braunschweig 1978).

20. Möhr, J.R., Haehn, K.D., Dreibholz, K.J.: Analysis and Stand-
    ardization of the Activities of the General Practitioner in
    Preparation for a Computeroriented Information System. In
    Anderson, J. and Forsythe, J.M. (Eds.): MEDINFO 74, pp. 453 -
    457. (North Holland Publ. Co., Amsterdam 1974).

21. Möhr, J.R., Haehn, K.D. (Hrsg.): Verdenstudie - Strukturanalyse
    allgemeinmedizinischer Praxen. Schriftenreihe des Zentralin-
    stituts für die kassenärztliche Versorgung in der Bundesrepublik
    Deutschland, Wiss. Reihe, Bd. 7. (Deutscher Ärzteverlag,
    Köln 1977).

22. Niedersächsisches Landesverwaltungsamt - Statistik-: Bevölkerung
    der Gemeinden am 30. Juni 1976. Statistische Berichte.
    (Hannover 1976).

23. Petrowsky, A.M.: Systems Analysis of Some Bio-Medical Problems
    Related to Medical Treatment Management. (International
    Institute for Applied Systems Analysis, IIASA Publication RM-75-
    23, Laxenburg 1975).

24. Reichertz, P.L.: Hospitals and Health Care. IFAC 75, 6th Tri-
    ennial World Congress of the International Federation of Auto-
    matic Control, Boston/Mass./USA, Aug. 20-30, 1975, p7.1-p7.23.
    (Instrument Society of America, Pittsburg, Pa. 1975).

25. Reichertz, P.L., Möhr, J.R., Holthoff, G., Filsinger, E.:
    Struktur und Funktion der allgemeinmedizinischen Praxis. Ergeb-
    nisse einer Analyse zur Untersuchung der Grundlagen für Computer-
    unterstützung der allgemeinmedizinischen Praxis. Projekt-
    zwischenbericht. (Zentralinstitut für die kassenärztliche Ver-
    sorgung in der Bundesrepublik Deutschland, Köln 1976).

26. Reichertz, P.L.: Health Care Delivery as a System. In Reichertz,
    P.L. and Goos, G. (Eds.): Informatics and Medicine, pp. 32-54.
    (Springer, Heidelberg 1977).

27. Reichertz, P.L., Anderson, J.: A System View of Health Care
    Organizations. In Laudet, M., Anderson, J., Begon, F. (Eds.):
    Medical Computing, Proceedings of an International Symposium,
    Toulouse, March 22-25, 1977, pp. 87-98. (Taylor & Francis,
    London 1977).

28. Reichertz, P.L., Möhr, J.R., v. Gärtner-Holthoff, G., Schwarz, B.:
    Structural Analysis of General Practices in Lower Saxony.
    First World Conference on Mathematics at the Service of Man,
    Barcelona/Spain, July 11-16, 1977. (In press: Lecture Notes in
    Medical Informatics, Springer, Heidelberg).

29. Reichertz, P.L.: EDV und das System der Gesundheitsversorgung.
    In Reichertz, P.L., Schwarz, B. (Eds.): Informationssysteme in
    der Gesundheitsversorgung - Ökologie der Systeme. Verhandl.
    21. Jahrestag GMDS, 1976, S. 1-13. (Schattauer, Stuttgart 1978).

30. Reichertz, P.L., v. Gärtner-Holthoff, G., Möhr, J.R., Schwarz, B.:
    Struktur und Funktion der allgemeinmedizinischen Praxis. Studie
    in Niedersachsen 1977. Schriftenreihe des Zentralinstituts für
    die kassenärztliche Versorgung in der Bundesrepublik Deutschland,
    Wiss. Reihe, Bd. 10 (Deutscher Ärzteverlag, Köln 1978).

31. Reichertz, P.L., Möhr, J.R., Schwarz, B., Schlatter, A., von
    Gärtner-Holthoff, G., Filsinger, E.: Evaluation of a Field Test
    of Computers for the Doctor's Office. Meth. Inform. Med. 18
    (1979) 61-70.

I N D E X

List of Speakers

John Anderson, M.D.
Professor of Medicine
King's College Hospital Medical School
(University of London)
Denmark Hill
London, SE5 8RX
U.K.

Morris F. Collen, M.D.
Director
Department of Medical Methods Research
The Permanente Medical Group
3700 Broadway
Oakland, CA 94611
USA

Roger A. Côté, M.D.
Professor of Pathology
Faculty of Medicine
University of Sherbrooke
Sherbrooke, Quebec J1H-5N4
Canada

J. Malcolm Forsythe, M.D.
Regional Medical Officer
South East Thames
Regional Health Authority
Randolph House 46-48
Wellesley Road
Croydon CR9 3QA
U.K.

Sidney R. Garfield, M.D.
Kaiser Permanente Medical Care Program
Broadway
Oakland, CA 94611
USA

François Grémy, M.D.
Professor
Département de Biophysique et
Biomathématiques
Faculté de Médecine
Pitie Salpétrière
91, bd de l'Hôpital
F-75634 Paris Cedex 13
France

Gerd Griesser, Prof. Dr. med.
Präsident der
Christian-Albrechts-Universität zu Kiel
Olshausenstr. 40-60
D-2300 Kiel 1

Paul Hall, M.D.
Director
Multiphasic Health Test Center
Sophiahemmet
Box 5605
S-11486 Stockholm
Sweden

Shigekoto Kaihara, M.D.
Professor of Medical Informatics
Director, Hospital Computer Center
University of Tokyo Hospital
7 Hongo, Bunkyo-Ku T-113
Japan

Donald A.B. Lindberg, M.D.
Director
Information Science Group
University of Missouri-Columbia
School of Medicine
Lewis Hall
Columbia, Missouri 65211
USA

Gwilym S. Lodwick, M.D.
Professor of Radiology
University of Missouri
Medical Center
Columbia, Missouri 65201
USA

Ezio Masè, M.D.
President of Salutis Unitas
Via Tarvisio 5
I-00198 Roma
Italy

Hans Peterson, M.D.
Director
Stockholm County Council
Health Care Information System
Langholmsgatan 34-36
S-10270 Stockholm
Sweden

Peter L. Reichertz, Prof. Dr. med.
Department für Biometrie und Dokumentation
Abteilung für klinische Datenverarbeitung
und Dokumentation
Karl-Wiechert-Allee 9
D-3000 Hannover 61
F.R.G.

Angelo Serio, M.D.
Via Prisciana 26
I-00198 Roma
Italy

D.J. Shepley, M.D.
Whitby Clinic
200 Brock St North
Whitby, Ontario
Canada

Carlos Vallbona, M.D.
Professor of Community Medicine
Baylor College of Medicine
Houston, Texas 77025
USA

Gustav Wagner, Prof. Dr. med.
Director
Institute of Documentation,
Information and Statistics
The German Cancer Research Center
Im Neuenheimer Feld 280
D-6900 Heidelberg
F.R.G.

George Z. Williams, M.D., D.Sc.
Institute of Health Research
2200 Webster Street
San Francisco, CA 94115
USA

Medizinische Informatik und Statistik

Herausgeber: S. Koller, Mainz, P. L. Reichertz, Hannover, K. Überla, München

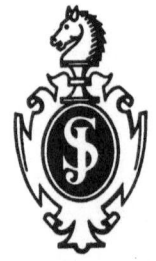

Springer-Verlag
Berlin
Heidelberg
New York